Nursing Civil Rights

WOMEN IN AMERICAN HISTORY

Editorial Advisors:
Susan K. Cahn
Deborah Gray White
Anne Firor Scott, Founding Editor Emerita

A list of books in the series appears at the end of this book.

Nursing Civil Rights

Gender and Race in the Army Nurse Corps

CHARISSA J. THREAT

UNIVERSITY OF ILLINOIS PRESS

Urbana, Chicago, and Springfield

Library of Congress Cataloging-in-Publication Data
Threat, Charissa J., 1976–
Nursing civil rights : gender and race in the Army Nurse Corps /
Charissa J. Threat.
pages   cm. — (Women, gender, and sexuality in American
history)
Includes bibliographical references and index.
ISBN 978-0-252-03920-1 (cloth : alk. paper)
ISBN 978-0-252-08077-7 (pbk. : alk. paper)
ISBN 978-0-252-09724-9 (e-book)
1. United States. Army Nurse Corps—History. 2. United States.
Army—Nurses—History—20th century. 3. Military nursing—
United States—History—20th century. 4. African American
women—History—20th century. 5. Male nurses—United States—
History—20th century. 6. Discrimination in employment—
United States—History—20th century. 7. Civil rights—United
States—History—20th century. 8. Sex role in the work
environment—United States—History—20th century. 9. World
War, 1939–1945—Participation, African American. 10. World
War, 1939–1945—Women—United States.
I. Title. II. Title: Gender and race in the Army Nurse Corps.
UH493.T57   2015
355.3'45—dc23   2014042894

To my sister Channa for support that knows no bounds.
And to my mother Jackie and brother Calvin.

Contents

Acknowledgments

Certainly, the saying "it takes a village" holds true for many things in life, and no less for the completion of a book. While the work of a historian is often solitary, it is by no means without a large group of family, friends, and colleagues to help move a project along. I am going to try my best not to forget to acknowledge all those without whose support this book would never have been completed.

I was quite fortunate to complete the work upon which this book is based under the direction of Leslie Schwalm at the University of Iowa. She is, without a doubt, an amazing mentor, advisor, and friend who believed in this project from the beginning and whose constant support, intellectual and otherwise, made this possible. I owe Johanna Schoen my gratitude for her generous reading of every aspect of the drafts and proposals on this subject. I would be remiss if I did not also thank two early mentors in my academic career, Fredrik Logevall, who eons ago, when I was an undergraduate at UCSB, stirred my interest on the topic of army nurses; and to Mary Farmer-Kaiser, who, as a young junior faculty member at University of Louisiana—Lafayette, took on a master's student without fear.

I am indebted to a long list of wonderful colleagues and friends who read this material, helped me hone the project, participated on various panels with me, kept me sane, plied me with food and drink, and always managed to make me smile through the craziness. I owe a special thanks to my colleagues and amazing writing group at the University of Iowa, who helped me frame and reframe my arguments and ideas over the course of too many years: Christy Clark-Pujara, Sharon Romeo, Karissa Haugeberg, Megan Threlkeld, John

McKerley, and Cari Campbell. I would also like to acknowledge my gratitude to Kara Dixon Vuic, Christine Knauer, Kimberly Jensen, Katherine Luongo, and Carol-Ann Farkas for giving generously of their time in reading material, asking questions, and providing wonderful intellectual sounding boards.

My readers at the University of Iowa Press, including Susan Malka and my anonymous reader, were quite generous in their advice and questions. Their suggestions have made this book better than I could have hoped. Thank you as well to my editor, Laurie Matheson, copyeditor Julie Gay, and the rest of the support team at the University of Illinois Press; they have made the publishing process smooth and seamless.

This book would have not been possible without the tremendous amount of help I received from the staff at a number of archives and libraries, including the Case Western Historical Society; Moorland-Spingarn Research Center at Howard University; the Army Nurse Corps Archives and a series of amazing ANC archivists who answered all my questions and graciously allowed me access to their records; and Diane Gallagher at the Howard Gotlieb Archival Research Center's Nursing Archives and Richard Barry at the ANA head-quarters, both of whom have taken the time and energy to help me navigate the massive ANA collection. I would also like to acknowledge the financial support I received in the process of completing this project, including support from the Graduate College and the History Department at the University of Iowa, and the History Department at Northeastern University.

Finally, working on a book requires not only endless support but also good-natured patience from family members; I am eternally grateful for a large extended family for keeping me grounded throughout the completion of this work. My dear extended family, Maria Donaire-Cirsovius and Ruediger Cirsovius, Ray and Evie Christian, Christy and Jesil Pujara, Kate Luongo, Rebecca Cronin, Heitiare, Tina, Jay, and the rest of my California family. Tom and Ebba Schoonover always believed I could do it and are two of the most wonderful grandparents and mentors a person could be lucky enough to have in this life. And to my mother, Jackie St. Germain; my stepfather, Steve St. Germain; my brother Calvin Threat; and my twin sister Channa Threat—thank you all for loving me and caring for me throughout the years.

Abbreviations

ANA	American Nurses' Association
ANC	Army Nurse Corps
NAACP	National Association for the Advancement of Colored People
NACGN	National Association of Colored Graduate Nurses
NLNE	National League for Nursing Education
NNCWS	National Nursing Council for War Service
NOPHN	National Organization for Public Health Nursing
SGO	Surgeon General's Office

Introduction

In the spring of 2000, the third African American female chief of the Army Nurse Corps (ANC) was informed that the first male nurse had been nominated as her replacement. In response, Brigadier General Bettye H. Simmons wrote, "The diversity of our members has made us smarter as an organization and stronger as a Corps."[1] Her comments to active-duty and retired nurses celebrated this promotion as a sign of the strength and progressiveness of the Army Nurse Corps. Nearly one hundred years after its founding, the ANC could claim a race and gender diversity between its membership and leadership that remained elusive in both the civilian nursing population and among the other branches of the military.[2] Simmons's comments, however, disclosed little about the historic relationship between the Army Nurse Corps and the movements for social justice during the twentieth century.

The mid-twentieth-century campaigns to integrate the U.S. Army Nurse Corps were part of a larger civil rights struggle. Between the early twentieth century and the war in Vietnam, African American female nurses and white male nurses labored simultaneously to re-imagine standard ideas of nurses as white and female. While not a unified movement, the push by both African American female and white male nurses for access to and participation in the U.S. Army Nurse Corps employed the language of "rights" and "discrimination." These efforts attracted race rights' advocates and organizations such as national civil rights leader Walter White and the National Association for the Advancement of Colored People (NAACP) who saw in the campaign to end the discriminatory practices of the ANC an additional space to reach for racial justice.

White male nurses complicate this story of racial civil rights by broadening the movement in two distinct ways. First, the addition of white male nurses suggests a need to expand not only the actors in, but also the breadth of, the civil rights movement. The inclusion of white men in a story seemingly about racial discrimination provides a space for scholars to push the boundaries of discrimination history, specifically with regard to who is and who is not included in that charge. While the quest for racial equality is the outward impetus of the movement, examining the civil rights struggle from the perspective of and struggle for economic independence, opportunity, and equality in employment broadens our understanding of the movement to include economic rights under the equal rights umbrella. Nancy MacLean's work on economic equality and Alice Kessler-Harris's work on economic citizenship provide some foundation for this assertion. Additionally, Susan Hirsch's work on the struggles at the Pullman Company at midcentury remind us that sex and race had long divided workplace environment and job opportunities—with the most lucrative opportunities set aside for white men—and so workplaces have therefore been spaces to examine discrimination and equality.[3] Using these and similar works as a foundation, this book arises from the premise that nursing, an occupation traditionally sex- and race-typed white and female, provides a place to examine how gender identities and racial ideologies are contested in mid-twentieth century American society. Both African American female and white male nurses demanded the right as trained professionals to have equal access and opportunity to work and earn a wage as nurses with comparable skills.

Second, these parallel campaigns reveal how gender ideologies served both to support and to hinder the civil rights movement. By gender, I refer to the socially constructed ideals that define the roles or behaviors, and the obligations of individuals based on biological sex difference.[4] This includes the feminine and masculine expectations that defined normative understandings of womanhood and manhood in the United States. As R. W. Connell argues, masculinity does not exist except in relation to femininity, and vice versa.[5] To varying degrees both groups of nurses and their supporters employed gender identities as a means of garnering support to end the restrictive policies of the ANC and the Army Medical Department. These efforts occurred as the nation witnessed a continuous period of instability, from international war emergencies to domestic social upheavals that redefined the social fabric of

American society; public debates about military nursing reflected wartime and Cold War exigencies.

The experiences of African American female and white male nurses reveal a different type of civil rights story. Their campaigns suggest that the civil rights struggles of the twentieth century did not always follow an uncomplicated, progressive arc toward social justice. Instead, these struggles had both progressive and conservative elements in challenging and reaffirming social hierarchies and patterns of discrimination. They depended on a constant negotiation of the meanings and privileges attached to race and gender. The integration campaigns were progressive in challenging artificial distinctions about men and women, white and African American capacities to nurse and have access to care. In this way the campaigns helped break down barriers in both the military and civilian nursing profession. They reveal the connection between political, economic, social, and cultural changes in American society and the evolution of nursing from an occupation in the late nineteenth century to a profession in the latter twentieth century.

The integration campaigns were also conservative. This study reveals how agents of change became defenders of exclusionary practices when some of the same women who challenged their exclusion from the military or civilian nursing profession, or those who had gained considerable status within the profession, were unwilling to extend the opportunities to men who sought out military nursing careers. Here, gender expectations that demarcated certain jobs as male or female remained stubbornly inflexible as some women, regardless of their race, expected and even encouraged nursing to remain largely the responsibility of women. On the other hand, as World War II expanded military service opportunities to women, white male nurses expected nursing to be an additional area where they could serve their country. The fact that this did not occur during the war or in its immediate aftermath uncovers the difficulties faced by men who trained to do what many understood to be a woman's job.

This study links the story of the Army Nurse Corps to critical events in the United States between World War II and the Vietnam War. First, it enables us to explore how war and wartime expectations shape activism and citizenship obligations within a specific historic circumstance. Historians have long suggested that the events and climates surrounding World War II acted as catalysts for change among women, particularly white, middle-class women. Moreover, as Linda Kerber demonstrated, military service has, since its founding, shaped citizenship obligations in the United States.

The integration campaigns by African American female and white male nurses suggest that World War II and conflicts arising during the postwar period provided multiple groups with the opportunity to use military service to challenge gender conventions and race discrimination. When drafting women for nursing service became a possibility during World War II, African American female nurses, for example, emphasized their sex—thus, their appropriateness to nurse—to challenge racial discrimination in the ANC. White male nurses, in contrast, argued that their sex should not hinder their ability to participate as nurses during the war and should, in fact, be welcomed in combat areas deemed too dangerous for women.[6]

Second, this study underscores the connection between the campaigns to integrate the ANC and the domestic and international anxieties during the Cold War by suggesting that anticommunism both hindered and supported the prospect for gender and race equality within the ANC and, by extension, civilian society.[7] The effort by male nurses to gain acceptance into the ANC during the 1950s—and, later, the struggle by female army nurses to gain benefits and change policies regarding their employment in the nurse corps—are set within the larger context of civilian society and the civilian nursing profession. Cold War anxieties, as well as domestic civil rights struggles, influenced the civilian nursing profession. In the postwar period nurse advocacy groups such as the American Nurses' Association (ANA) prioritized an antidiscrimination campaign in their bid to provide the nation with the best healthcare. This campaign not only reflected the influence of the civil rights movement on the nursing profession but also resulted in the civilian nursing profession extending its antidiscrimination goals toward modernizing and changing the ANC.

Third, this study departs from conventional gender narratives that focus solely on women in wartime and during the Cold War period in order to highlight how gender informed and was informed by war, social justice struggles, and economic independence. The effort on the part of male nurses demonstrates how one group of men challenged normative understandings of traditional gender roles by campaigning for acceptance into the military and into the ANC as nurses. Female nurses also used common assumptions about the tie between intimate care and femininity to promote their goals and resist the addition of male nurses. Within the context of social change during the mid-twentieth century, the campaigns to integrate the ANC both undermined and supported traditional gender expectations. The male nurse campaign and the female nurse response to it challenges how scholars traditionally understood the search for equity.[8] It expands the discussion on equality by suggesting that white men also had a space to push for economic equity and opportunity, while revealing some of the arguments women used to confirm their positions in nursing and the military.

Finally, for most of the twentieth century the historic link between social perceptions of what were believed to be women's biological abilities and the intimate setting of caregiving encouraged the public and the occupation's leadership to define nursing as a female "profession." As the occupation gained in stature, women of color were excluded as part of the process of professionalizing nursing, and as racial exclusivity further increased the status of white nurses, it became a largely white female occupation. These realities make the nursing profession an important location to examine and unearth the complex layers of interlocking interactions of gender and race in twentieth-century American society. Male nurses challenged both the gender bias of the profession and the popular acceptance of the notion that biological sex confirmed special traits necessary for nursing professionals. African American women also challenged the nursing profession's racial bias—especially the notion that women's "special" capabilities as nurses were racially exclusive to white womanhood—and used nursing to pursue larger claims to equality. In the context of World War II, the Cold War, and conflicts in Asia, this study uses the microcosm of military nursing to illuminate contests over race and gender discrimination and social justice. It reveals that the U.S. military, especially in the period between World War II and the Vietnam War, was a reflection of the social and cultural values of American society, not divided from them. The experiences of white and African American female nurses in the ANC and the push for male integration throughout the 1940s, 1950s, and 1960s reveal that changes in policy did not alter practices of discrimination and inequality.[9]

This book investigates claims to the title of nurse during the peak decades of contestation by both African American and white women, and, later, white men who fought for recognition within the civilian and military nursing profession. It exposes the nursing profession's role in larger conversations about gender roles and identities, racial equality, and economic opportunity. Excluded from medical schools through practices of gender discrimination, women claimed nursing as a "profession" where popular notions of female attributes were valuable assets. The professionalization of the occupation was a process however, one that pitted the leadership's vision of the profession, which included membership in professional associations, training in acceptable degree programs, and licensure, against individual nurses and a male-dominated, medical-establishment's vision of nursing as a female occupation and obligation. Regardless, I will use the term nurse, trained nurse, and registered nurse interchangeably to indicate those nurses who obtained both advanced training and a state license, as it was these nurses for whom the ANC limited acceptance, and it was largely male nurses who fit this criteria who wanted to join the ANC. Furthermore, while nursing scholars generally agree that nursing became a true profession—defined by university education and advanced degrees—in the 1960s and 1970s, I will use the terms "nursing profession" and "professional nursing" to represent nursing as an occupation within a specific historic moment—that is, nursing as part of a cadre of "women's professions" that emerged near the end of the nineteenth century and were seen as acceptable work for white, middle- and upper-class women and as an avenue for upward mobility and respectability for working-class white and nonwhite women. The terms "profession" or "professional" were used by nursing leaders and some nurses as a way to improve the stature of the occupation, not to suggest that nursing was a profession in the same way as doctors or lawyers in the early twentieth century. Furthermore, these terms and titles were often bestowed on nurses and the occupation by the communities in which they lived and worked and by individuals they helped, as a mark of respect.[10]

An examination of institutional, organizational, and personal sources reveals the civil rights story of the Army Nurse Corps. Institutional records at the Army Nurse Corps Archives and the National Archives and Records Administration expose a persistent dialogue between the military authority, nurses, and civilians concerning the recruitment and responsibility of army nurses. Much of the material gleaned from these two locations reveals official discussions about the daily functioning of the Army Nurse Corps and nurses within the army medical structure. Read in conjunction with newspaper accounts, personal correspondence, and early histories of military nursing, administrative records reveal the complexity and, at times, contradictory nature of military nursing. For example, records about the founding of the ANC disclose how the race and gender biases of the profession's white leaders shaped early ANC policies that defined members as white and female.[11] At the same time, documents from the U.S. Army and National Archives disclose that nursing shortages and wartime needs challenged this identity and resulted in a recurring debate about who qualified to be a military nurse. Wartime emergencies provided opportunities for black and even white women and white men to challenge restrictive policies in the ANC and restrictive nursing customs generally.

Organizational records from the National Association of Colored Graduate Nurses (NACGN), the NAACP, and the ANA help construct a narrative of the social justice challenges permeating the ANC during the mid-twentieth century. Yet as with the administrative records of the U.S. Army and ANC, these required reading the sources as one part of the larger story. The records kept by these organizations—and even gaining access to the full records of the organizations—influenced the story of the relationship between these groups and the ANC. Finally, individual and personal sources—where available— such as letters, diaries, and personal accounts about nursing experiences speak about attempts to breech barriers in the ANC by nurses and nurse advocates. They also unearth a much-needed picture of the lived experiences of some minority nurses within the profession.[12]

Chapter 1 focuses on the early evolution of nursing from the mid-nineteenth century through the early twentieth century. As it evolved, nursing care became both gendered and racialized in civilian society. Nursing's tie to intimate care meant that the early profession and its participants were cognizant of the values and beliefs surrounding gender roles and race relations that permeated social relationships and interactions in civilian society. This shaped who was a nurse and how nursing care was provided to those in need. War and military nursing needs played a large role in shaping the evolution of the modern nursing profession. Florence Nightingale's work during the Crimean War had a profound influence on changing nursing and preventative care in Western society; however, this chapter points to the Civil War as the transformative moment in the history of nursing in the United States, moving nursing from an unpaid obligation to a paid occupation. Late-nineteenth-century perceptions of nursing effortlessly transferred to the military at the turn of the twentieth century as the U.S. Congress passed the Army Reorganization Act of 1901, which founded the Army Nurse Corps.

Chapters 2 and 3 examine the efforts by black female nurses and white male nurses to claim a space for themselves in a profession that relegated them to the margins. Chapter 2 explores the World War II integration campaign by African American female nurses. It traces how African American female nurses came to understand the importance of their campaign within the larger context of a civil rights campaign from the late 1930s through World War II. In an effort to break down racial barriers, however, African American nurses successfully co-opted traditional gender conventions to make the claim that the sex of the nurse, not race, should determine nursing care for soldiers. This focus on gender roles and responsibilities, especially in the latter half of the war, when the U.S. military and federal government debated the drafting of female nurses, resulted in the successful end to race restrictions in the ANC but helped perpetuate a gender bias against male nurses.

Chapter 3 asserts that World War II also provided an opportunity for male nurses to mount a campaign to integrate the ANC as part of their larger strategy for equality within the nursing profession. Less organized than African American female nurses, male nurses nonetheless made claims for inclusion and recognition in the military nurse corps based on their training. Furthermore, race discrimination in the nursing profession revealed that this campaign was largely a story of white male nurses; little information about minority male nurses exists. This unusual set of circumstances exposes a shared history of discrimination between African American female and white male nurses. While national calls for nurses remained unrelenting before and during the war, male nurses made little progress in challenging the understanding that the profession, both civilian and military, was a female occupation and duty. In fact, the proposed drafting of women nurses during the war reinforced this understanding as both opponents of the *Nurse Draft Bill* and civil rights activists stressed that there were female nurses available for service, but whom the military had rejected based on race. While scholars often argue that race had the preeminent function in shaping social roles and perceptions, the male nurse campaign during World War II reveals how gender and biological sex could transcend race.

Chapters 4 and 5 follow the integration campaign during the postwar period and within the context of the Cold War and the expanding civil rights movement. Chapter 4 uncovers how worries about national security shaped the Army Nurse Corps' response to male nurse integration and the push to desegregate the U.S. military. It reveals that while the civilian nursing profession promoted—at least on the surface—equality and fair opportunity for its members as part of their defense mission, the ANC reinforced its gendered opinion on nursing within the nurse corps. Female nurse officers encouraged the continued gender delineation in nursing as a way to protect their autonomy and position within the ANC. In the wake of the Korean War, male nurses realized a significant accomplishment in their acceptance into the Reserve Officers Corps, signaling a measure of military recognition of male nurses. It was war, both literal and figurative, that placed the ANC in a position that helps scholars understand how Cold War fears, postwar life and stability, and social-justice challenges collide.

Chapter 5 addresses the Army Nurse Corps' attempt to deal with not only civil rights activism but also women's rights and gender equality in a fast-changing society. Years after the 1948 mandate of nondiscrimination in the U.S. military and the 1955 integration of male nurses, conservative race and gender beliefs challenged progressive attempts at social justice. The ANC provides the perfect microcosm for examining the complexities and contradictions of "equality" in the late 1950s and 1960s. The aggressive shift in the civil rights movement, a growing women's rights movement, conversations about an equal rights amendment, and the war in Vietnam radically transformed the ways Americans understood gender and racial hierarchies. The ANC's struggles to alleviate ongoing nursing shortages are juxtaposed with a civil society in social flux and a military engaged in yet another Asian war. These struggles uncover the differences between individual and institutional experiences, as well as policy changes at the organizational level in much the same way that the 1954 *Brown v. Board of Education* decision and later the 1964 Civil Rights Act revealed in the search for racial equality. Changing military policies regarding the race and sex of military nurses reveal a recurring negotiation between traditional race and gender relationships and shifting cultural norms.

Finally, the conclusion offers insight into how the integration campaigns and the history of the ANC over a thirty-year period help scholars understand a more inclusive civil rights story and the evolution of nursing into a modern profession in the latter part of the twentieth century. While the army, and by extension the ANC, remained stoically committed to distancing themselves from the social upheavals and social-justice activities taking place in civil society, in reality they often found themselves at the forefront of these conversations and campaigns. At the same time, as civilian nurse training and education shifted to university baccalaureate degrees, graduate schools, and advanced specialty programs, these changes also made their mark on the ANC. As the Vietnam War reached its peak in the late 1960s, gender and racial tensions remained. The 1966 admittance of male nurses to the regular army did not diminish the scrutiny faced by men who served or wanted to serve as nurses. Furthermore, the army continued to grapple with recruitment and retention of minority nurses as well, even facing charges of race discrimination at the Walter Reed Army Institute of Nursing in the early 1970s.

1

The Politics of Intimate Care

Gender, Race, and Nursing Work

The nascent reality of nurses as trained professionals found an audience amid the evolution of the medical profession during the 1850s in Europe and the United States. As the field of medicine became more sophisticated and developed—focusing on preventative care and not just healing—so, too, did ideas about patient care and who had the authority to provide and control that care. With "professionalization," medical authority became gendered. Society viewed men as having both the intellectual and physical capabilities necessary for the medical profession.[1] In contrast, as the fairer sex, women were seen as fragile, weak, and lacking in the brain capacity necessary to successfully attend to medical emergencies. In addition, late-nineteenth-century Victorian notions of sexual propriety made such work unsuitable for women.[2] The increasingly male-dominated medical profession strongly opposed women entering professionalized medicine, even as nurse leaders attempted to professionalize their occupation. In a 1904 address titled "The Nurse and the Medical Man," Dr. Casey Wood described the job differences between doctor and nurse as the "practice of medicine and the art of nursing." Doctors in the late nineteenth and early twentieth century agreed that the "success of the physician's treatment" went hand in hand with the help of a cooperative, loyal, and obedient nurse, but many doctors did not view nursing as a scientific profession, nor could they envision nursing as an autonomous profession.[3] Exacerbating this viewpoint was the fact that until the 1870s, the hospital remained only a peripheral institution for the medical care of most individuals, a place most went to die, and nursing occurred primarily within the confines of domestic responsibility, as both duty and obligation provided by women for their families and neighbors. Therefore, as Dr. Wood's comments suggest, nursing performed outside of the home needed the careful and expert supervision of doctors to find success in the professional world.

By the turn of the twentieth century, nursing moved from an unpaid domestic obligation for "respected" ladies or paid labor employing undesirable women, to the paid occupation of respectable working women.[4] As one of several "women's professions," nursing particularly attracted white, middle- and upper-class women, among whom the first training schools actively recruited. For these women, the opening of schools of nursing imbued nursing with a semi-professional status, one that provided nurses with "a type of public stature and power previously reserved for men."[5] Nevertheless, nurses walked a fine line, one that meant reimagining nursing in a way that did not completely negate the domestic "art" vision many had of respectable vocations for women outside the home. Women began promoting this activity as both duty and responsibility to family and community, and late-nineteenth-century war and warfare provided the medium.[6] Beginning with the Civil War, wartime exigencies allowed women to co-opt nursing as female work. Wartime relief work—exemplified most concisely with nurses—became the catalyst for change, particularly for white women. Military nursing, in particular, promoted the formalization of the nursing practice.

War and wartime experiences are entwined with the history and meaning of nursing in the United States. Here, what were understood as female obligation (caregiving) and male duty (soldiering) are juxtaposed with the reality of need. The history of the Army Nurse Corps (ANC) is rife with examples of how war complicates social, cultural, and economic beliefs and values that organized and informed American society. Just as military participation has historically defined citizenship and access to the rights that go along with it, military nursing also challenged notions of who had rights, the types of rights, and access to them through military service. A focus on the ANC and its nurses helps to illuminate the relationship between the military and civilian populace, revealing trends in nursing practices, debates about work, and concerns about war taking place in the larger civil society. In this sense, the transformation of nursing—from paid occupation in the late nineteenth century to autonomous profession within the medical field during the second half of the twentieth century—suggests not only that "gender informs work" but that work was transformed by "existing relationships of power and inequality" as well as changing social, economic, and cultural conditions.[7]

War, Women, and Modern Nursing

In the fall of 1854, Florence Nightingale—an upper-class woman from an influential English family—lead a group of women nurses to the Crimean War front. The British assigned Nightingale the task of resolving the deplorable health and sanitary conditions that were crippling the British Army. Nightingale, who trained as a nurse against her family's wishes, challenged the popular images of nursing as uncouth work. Instead, she set out to "correct the evils in nursing," and starting in the mid-1840s trained and educated herself and others with this in mind.[8] She believed that healthcare, in the form of sanitary knowledge rather than a medical degree, resulted in a healthier population. In many ways, Dr. Wood's comments about the "art of nursing" reinforced Nightingale's earlier vision of nursing. Further, Nightingale asserted that health encompassed not only diet but also cleanliness and environment; this was something that the medical profession was also beginning to recognize in the same period. The combination of all three prevented disease and ensured a quick recovery from ailment.

In late October 1854 Nightingale arrived in the Crimea to conditions that participants later described as the source of nearly three-quarters of the casualties suffered by the British.[9] In the time between her arrival and the end of the Crimean War in early 1856, Nightingale's reorganization of British military hospitals throughout Crimea—including the institution of basic sanitary, dietary, and social services for soldiers—resulted in an astonishing overall drop in the mortality rate from 42 percent to 2.2 percent.[10] Yet despite her success, particularly in advancing the idea that respectable women had a place within the medical profession, Nightingale and the nursing occupation faced large obstacles in the male-dominated medical community.

Most men, at least initially, resented Nightingale's meddling as an outsider and worried about the results of her intrusion. In what became a recurring theme into the twentieth century, female nurses—especially those who participated during military conflicts—had to contend with resentment from many male medical professionals, especially doctors, and anger over the possibility that women nurses would ultimately undermine military authority.[11] Yet Nightingale's success during the Crimean War did champion nursing as a respectable female occupation, and her reforms became the foundation for the professionalization of nursing in both England and the United States. Nightingale's activities in the Crimean War enabled her to gain enough financial support to open the first nurse training schools for women in Britain, and although she warned women not to be involved in medical politics, she politicized and identified herself and women as the only authorities on nursing in the medical profession.[12]

The experiences and work of Nightingale and her female nurses resonated with many in the United States. Adequate care for soldiers was a recurring concern for U.S. military officials with each successive conflict in American history since the Revolutionary War. Until the Civil War, however, the role of the nurse was unorganized, and nursing—especially military nursing— was a loosely defined occupation. Hospital and battlefield work was the domain of men. The role of the domestic caregiver, as nursing was traditionally understood, remained the purview of women.[13] Throughout the Civil War, temporary volunteer or short-term staffing by men and women met all nursing needs in the military. This raised few questions, therefore, about either defining the profession of nursing or the parameters of nurse care. Nurses came from a multitude of backgrounds that included men, women, and minorities, as well as Catholic nuns and individuals from other religious orders, and until the late nineteenth century nurses were known by a variety of titles, including hospital stewards, nurse matrons, or surgeons' mates. Their duties included basic sanitary and domestic work such as housekeeping and ward keeping; they served as cooks or dieticians, and laundresses.

The evolution of nursing from volunteer obligation to paid work was a direct result of miscalculation in the first few months of the Civil War and the expectation of the conflict ending quickly. The unanticipated carnage during those first months of the war allowed for challenges to notions of gender- and class-appropriate behavior. Upper-class white women in the North, moved by a sense of patriotism and worry about loved ones, and working- and middle-class black and white women, realizing the possibilities of earning an income, joined military life among the Union Army through hospital and relief work.[14] This work appropriated idealized constructions of women's morality and "natural" caretaking abilities and tested the restrictions or limitations of a woman's proper place. Women argued that their proper place was wherever their natural abilities were needed. The participation of women in nursing and hospital work during the Civil War also provided the foundation for co-opting nursing as a white, female, and middle-class occupation in the years following the war.

Two Civil War policies and structural changes directly influenced women's participation in wartime activities and furthered the evolution of nursing.[15] First, in June 1861 the army commissioned the first superintendent of women nurses, Dorothea Dix. Already well known for her work with insane asylums, Dix had offered her services free of charge to organize military hospitals and supply female nurses during the first month of the war. Her services were accepted by the secretary of war (Union), and she became "responsible to select and assign women nurses . . . in military hospitals, [where] they not be employed without her sanction and approval, except in cases of urgent need."[16] In essence, Dix's commission as the first superintendent of an "army nurse corps" not only sanctioned women's presence in military hospitals but also defined the requirements of women who sought the title of "nurse" in public.

Under Dix's influence nurses were required to be "between the ages of thirty-five and fifty . . . and [have a] 'matronly' appearance," while also displaying "good conduct, or superior education, and serious disposition." Dix's strict requirements reflected her belief that only middle- and upper-class women, educated and from good families, could serve in this capacity.[17] The military and the white public concurred with Dix that only white women could meet the expectation of good conduct and respectability. While this was one avenue to gain official status with the medical department, women who did not fall into Dix's narrow parameters and wished to serve as nurses found other ways of doing so. Some women followed male loved ones, nursing with their regiments; other women joined relief organizations such as the United States Sanitary Commission (USSC) or were hired for domestic services and ultimately served as nurses.[18] Therefore, the contingent of women serving as nurses comprised both white and black women, working- and middle-class women, and elite women as well.[19]

The second change influencing women's participation in wartime activities—congressional passage of Public Order 38—granted women validation for their nursing service. Beginning in June 1861, the order provided some female nurses a wage of forty cents per day, or about twelve dollars a month for their labor.[20] This was an enormous opportunity for women. For those who could take advantage of the chance to earn an income, the pay provided women a way to experience economic independence and therefore some measure of control over both their public and private lives. Not all women, however, wanted a wage, and some women, particularly elite women, volunteering for nursing service were careful to set themselves apart from women who received wages.[21] Instead, they believed that their service as nurses was within the boundaries of their *duty* as respectable women; to receive a wage degraded that female obligation and those volunteers shouldering it.

By the end of the Civil War, nearly six thousand women served as nurses.[22] Yet, however celebrated women's participation within the military was, the U.S. Army viewed their positions as a temporary addition made in time of crisis. At the end of the conflict, the U.S. military terminated the employment of female nurses. Nursing for the Medical Department of the United States Army reverted to the domain of male soldiers. Most of the women relief workers returned to their prewar activities, and many would not participate in the nascent nursing profession or work in the medical field in any capacity following the Civil War.[23] For some, however, the foray into the wage-labor market as nurses was not over.

Men and the Early Practice of Nursing

Men have had a long, if unacknowledged, history in nursing under the auspices of both religious and military orders. Men founded many of the early Christian hospitals and institutions for the sick and infirm in Europe. Strict sex segregation of care, however, meant that both men and women staffed these institutions.[24] Monks and laymen took care of men in hospitals, while nuns and the traditional midwife cared for women in hospitals and homes.[25] Men also organized groups dedicated to nursing that eventually became religious orders, which until the sixteenth century were overwhelmingly male dominated. As early as 1095, a father and son founded the Hospital Brothers of St. Anthony in southeastern France. The original members were laymen, but by the thirteenth century members had taken monastic vows. Other religious nursing orders included the Brotherhood of Santo Spirito, the Alexian Brothers, and the Brothers of the Happy Death.[26] The existence of such orders reveals nursing as a much more diverse activity historically than is commonly known.

Religious orders were not the only institutions in which men focused on nursing as a function of their mission. Soldiering unarguably necessitated the need for nursing; consequently, beginning with the crusades of the eleventh century, military orders established branches to ensure the care of their soldiers. Members of these military orders frequently provided care and nursing for private citizens in their immediate surroundings as well.[27] While these orders changed over time, and nursing became a priority in the missions for some but not all, it was nonetheless a duty performed by male soldiers.[28] The histories of these military and religious nursing orders reveal the need to reevaluate the history of nursing. What accounted for the decline in men's participation and leadership in nursing to the point that the occupation became primarily associated with women's work, duty, and obligation?

Florence Nightingale's nursing reforms were certainly one factor in reconceptualizing the place of men in nursing. The number of men practicing nursing, however, was already on the decline by the time Nightingale pushed for nursing to become the domain of women inside and outside the home in the mid-nineteenth century. According to scholar Chad E. O'Lynn, three social changes contributed to the decline of men in nursing between the sixteenth and nineteenth centuries. The first was the decrease in monasteries and male military nursing orders and the increase of convents and female nursing orders during the Renaissance. Convents increased in scope and size as the number of women entering religious orders swelled. Women increasingly worked in hospitals and provided care for the sick as part of their religious life. Second, nursing became less organized and disciplined once the responsibility of nursing moved from religious to secular hospitals in the nineteenth century. Many scholars link this shift to the decline in the quality of nursing as oversight in the personnel who worked in secular hospitals was less organized. This change eventually gained infamy, as represented by Charles Dickens's literary character Sarah Gamp.[29] Finally, the social effects of the Industrial Revolution contributed significantly to the decline of men in nursing. The growth of factories and heavy industry required physical labor that employers deemed appropriate only for men. These jobs attracted men, O'Lynn argues, because they paid better wages than any farm or menial job and required no formal education.[30] The modest wages and unglamorous work of nursing held little appeal for men even during wartime and as part of military pursuits during the nineteenth century.

Nightingale's successful reduction of the British Army's mortality rate during the Crimean War persuaded U.S. military officials of the necessity of proper care for their own soldiers.[31] However, in keeping with mid-nineteenth-century ideas about gender roles, which excluded women among military ranks, the U.S. Army looked to its male soldiers, not female volunteers, to fill the role of nurse. In 1856, Congress authorized the recruitment of male soldiers as "hospital stewards for the care of the sick and wounded" within the U.S. Army Hospital Corps.[32] This cadre of male soldiers became a small, semi-permanent group attached to the army's Medical Department and a more consistent source of labor than had previously existed in the military. Although army records do not indicate the race of the hospital stewards, we have to assume that it was primarily white men who served within the Hospital Corps. Slavery and racism kept most African American and other minorities out of the U.S. Army even before the Civil War. Their duties included all manner of patient care, assisting surgeons and doctors in work that was similar to that carried out later by female nurses. Unlike the efficiency of Nightingale's nurses among the British Army during the

Crimean War, the employment of male soldiers as hospital stewards in the United States proved problematic almost from the beginning.

The hospital corps was an unattractive assignment for male soldiers. Many regarded the work associated with the assignment as menial, chores better suited to women than men. This included doing laundry, cleaning wards, and preparing meals for patients. The work also exposed the stewards to unsanitary conditions, including contact with infectious diseases. Furthermore, the low pay associated with this assignment made the hospital corps unappealing to many men. As one U.S. Surgeon General suggested, stewards needed "to look for their reward in heaven" because no such reward existed on earth. Congress agreed in 1856, stating that because the "laborious and loathsome duties they have to perform and in consideration of their frequent exposure to contagious diseases," stewards would receive thirty dollars per month plus extra pay. Nevertheless, even the extra pay was not enough to overcome the serious limitations in the organization and number of stewards. They eventually failed to meet the demands that arose during the Civil War.[33]

Within the first two months of the fighting between Union and Confederate forces, Union military officials realized that they needed extra nurses to supplement the hospital stewards. The war lasted longer than anyone predicted, so battlefield casualties escalated, and the relatively small number of stewards found themselves overwhelmed by the sick and wounded. Although men still contracted and worked as nurses, large numbers of women seized the opportunity to become directly involved in the hostilities by volunteering to care for the wounded. Under pressure from the United States Sanitary Commission, the War Department acquiesced to the employment of female nurses by formalizing their participation in the summer of 1861. As the war progressed, women came to dominate nursing care. Nevertheless, the Union Army and federal government did not view the service that female nurses provided in the same way they viewed the contribution of male stewards. This is most obvious in the compensation differences between male stewards and female nurses. Men who performed the "laborious and loathsome" duty of nursing received thirty dollars per month; compensation for women required a congressional order that provided a mere twelve dollars per month for those lucky enough to receive pay at all.[34]

By war's end, the work of female nurses and the vast number of women who participated in this capacity encouraged some middle- and upper-class female reformers in the United States to transform nursing into a legitimate and respectable occupation for their daughters. They had a prime model of this possibility with the nursing reforms and school of nursing Florence

Nightingale opened in London in 1860. Following her teachings, which included the belief that nursing was an activity best suited to women, American women pushed for the opening of training schools that supported Nightingale's particular vision of nursing. Male nurses, who once dominated the activity outside the home, were only minor players in this new profession. Indeed, if some nurse activists had their way, the budding profession would exclude men altogether.

Nurse Training Schools and the Gendering of the Profession

As Florence Nightingale's experience during the Crimean War shaped her belief in the necessity of training schools for female nurses, so too did the Civil War experiences influence the group of American women who went on to build nurse training schools for women in the United States. They saw training schools as Nightingale did, as both the method to ensure the best healthcare for people and the means of providing a respectable occupation—a means of self-support—for daughters of white working- and middle-class families.[35] A few hospitals began training schools for nursing early in the 1870s, the most notable being the New England Hospital for Women and Children in 1872. These hospital schools extended the mission of the hospitals and provided workers to care for patients. In 1873, three nurse-training schools opened in the Northeast, modeled on Nightingale's belief that "women should control the teaching and practice of nursing."[36] The first of these was the Bellevue Hospital School of Nursing in New York City. The opening of Bellevue and other training schools for women challenged the role of men in nursing; male nurses did not become extinct, but they became endangered.[37] Their opportunities, duties, and roles in the occupation were, increasingly, narrowly defined.

Nursing schools dedicated to training men did eventually open, but in far fewer numbers and more than ten years after the first schools opened for women. By that time nursing had already developed into a sex-segregated occupation. Women trained in general nursing, which taught them to assist doctors and attend male and female patients alike. In contrast, men trained to work in only two areas: in psychiatric hospitals, a role later known as psychiatric nursing, and in men's wards as male attendants. Nursing scholars traced these differences in education not only to contemporary ideals about gender roles but also to early employment of men in asylums in the late eighteenth and nineteenth centuries. Well into the twentieth century, supporters and opponents of men in nursing framed their arguments on physical differences and inherent biological traits. Asylums and psychiatric institutions needed male strength to deal with "the often violent and custodial nature of the work . . . and with strict segregation of the sexes," expressed one nurse on the place of men in the occupation. While another nurse wrote, "As a rule, I think the gentle touch of a women is more valuable to the sick than the greater strength of a man." This is not to suggest that there were no advocates supporting the equal training of young men and women in the occupation, but rather it reveals how the lack of uniform training between women and men from the foundation of the occupation in the United States rested largely on assumptions about biological capabilities and resulted in defining the title and responsibility of the nurse by sex.[38] This lack of uniform training between women and men and even among different groups of women served as the impetus for professionalization of the occupation during the twentieth century.[39]

The first training schools for men nurses opened between the 1880s and World War I.[40] In 1886 the McLean Hospital School of Nursing in Massachusetts opened its school to men and was one of the earliest training hospitals to accept both men and women. However, women received instruction in general nursing, including obstetric nursing, while men received instruction in "male genitourinary diseases" and trained to work in psychiatric wards.[41] Two years later, the Mills Training School for Men began training men to work in the men's wards of Bellevue Hospital, New York.[42] Eventually, the school merged with the Bellevue Hospital School of Nursing, and while briefly closed during World War II, it reopened again in 1948. The school is especially notable for its 1957 change in curriculum that allowed male nurses to study obstetrics.[43] The Alexian Brothers, a male Catholic religious order with a long history of nursing, had moved a branch of the group to the United States in the late nineteenth century and opened a hospital in Chicago in 1898 and then another in St. Louis in 1928. The Pennsylvania Hospital School of Nursing had an established history as a school for women when, on the eve of World War I, it decided to open a school for men at the Department of Mental and Nervous Diseases. LeRoy Craig, a male nurse who trained at the McLean School, directed the new institution. Believing in a more holistic approach to training male nurses, the school organized the curriculum to educate male nurses in a fashion similar to female nurses. Upon completion of their general course requirements, male nurses could then specialize in psychiatric and urological nursing.[44]

Even as schools of nursing for men expanded, male nurses remained a small minority in the occupation and an even smaller voice in the leadership of the nursing field. "Male nurse" became almost an oxymoron. Popular perception held that men who chose nursing did so because they were either unable to succeed as doctors or intended to use nursing as a stepping-stone to other pursuits in the medical profession. Certainly, this defined the experiences of some male nurses, but not all. Nevertheless, as the profession evolved and nursing specialties developed, a number of male nurses pursued specialties that required more training and were often more technical than general nursing. Intentional or not, some of these sub-specialties accentuate characteristics that define gender behaviors associated specifically with men or women. One of the best examples of this in the twentieth century is in the field of anesthesia, a specialty that a significant number of men found attractive not only for its technical requirements but for its reliance on self-sufficiency.[45] Registered nurses who wished to train as nurse anesthetists completed additional coursework that included everything from physiology and anatomy to pharmacology and anesthesia. In the early 1900s, this required an additional six months of education; by the end of the twentieth century, the requisite coursework spanned three years. Yet, as one contemporary male nurse recalled with regard to his choice of the nurse anesthetist specialty, "I still wanted to go into medicine, some field that would give me the opportunity for some independence."[46]

What defined nursing at the advent of the twentieth century was a nascent profession led and dominated by women and defined as female, with the exception of specific subspecialties. The trained nurse—labeled "registered nurse" and "graduate nurse" upon successfully passing state license exams—became the demarcation that reflected standing and wage-earning potential among nurses.[47] Along with membership in a national professional association such as the American Nurses' Association, this delineation helped nursing leaders establish a hierarchy as they moved the occupation toward professionalization. However, gender politics and racial practices banned outright or restricted men and nonwhite women from most training schools and professional nursing associations. White female nursing leaders had effectively reduced the opportunities for black women and white men to claim the title of professional nurse in its earliest iteration.

Wartime Nursing Advances Battle Lines in the Profession

During the Spanish-American War, the U.S. Army once again acknowledged the need for a corps of nurses. Soldiers training in the southern United States experienced outbreaks of typhoid, malaria, and other epidemic diseases. The responsibility of taking care of ill soldiers overwhelmed the army. Faced with this dilemma, the army had no choice but to contract with civilian nurses, but the contract nurse of 1898 was vastly different from her counterpart of the Civil War. Two decades had passed since the opening of the first nurse training schools. Additionally, by 1898 trained nurses prepared to join the U.S. Army well outside the domestic home front, in places like Cuba, the Philippines, and Hawaii.

The immense task of selecting and organizing women to join the army fell to Anita Newcomb McGee, a prominent Washington, D.C., physician and member of the Daughters of the American Revolution. McGee and her committee chose trained female nurses based on three criteria. First, recommendation letters from a physician and the head of the nurse's training school had to demonstrate the nurse's "professional ability." Second, the committee sought confirmation of the nurse's "moral character and reputation," in the form of a letter from a citizen of good standing in her community. Finally, a nurse had to prove her good health. Although McGee's requirements for contract nurses were stringent, rampant epidemics provided the opportunity for a small group of men, Catholic nuns, and African American women to contract as nurses during the war.[48] For example, an outbreak of yellow fever had McGee searching for nurses who were resistant to the disease. Of the eighty African American women she employed, thirty-two of them were resistant to yellow fever. By August 1898, the army contracted with about twelve hundred women to serve as nurses, and by the end of the three-month war, fifteen hundred women had participated.[49]

Despite the short duration of the Spanish-American War, the army did not automatically annul all nursing contracts as it had after the Civil War. Instead, roughly two hundred female contract nurses chose voluntarily to remain in service with the army, acting as a reserve supply of nurses when the next emergency arose. The army could no longer deny what trained nurses could do for its Medical Department, but it was not quite ready for women as a permanent part of its organization. Still, the military recognized that the presence of trained female nurses resulted in the decrease of deaths from disease and injury. Moreover, according to a number of reports, female nurses helped increase the "morale of not only their patients, but of everyone around them." This narrative became an important aspect of the arguments for a permanent group of nurses attached to the military.[50]

The successful employment of trained female nurses led nurses and their advocates, which included McGee and other well-connected middle- and upper-class women, to pressure the army and Congress to establish a permanent nurse corps. In response to this well-organized campaign and in recognition of the service provided by nurses during the Spanish-American War, Congress passed the Army Reorganization Act of 1900, which allowed for the formation of the Army Nurse Corps (ANC). This was the first permanent nurse corps of women to exist in any branch of the U.S. military. Formalized in 1901 as an auxiliary of the U.S. Army Medical Corps, the ANC, as stipulated by the Reorganization Act, could be composed of women only.[51]

From the beginning, the ANC maintained a connection to the civilian nursing profession. The second superintendent of the ANC, Jane Delano, came to the military through her work with the American Red Cross and the Nurses Associated Alumnae.[52] Representatives from the army and the Army Nurse Corps would eventually serve on the board of directors or as members of committees for the American Nurses' Association, National Organization for Public Health Nursing, and the National League for Nursing Education. Additionally, the American Red Cross became responsible for the recruitment and enrollment of nurses in the Armed Forces Nurse Corps.[53] Civilian nursing and the ANC existed in a symbiotic relationship, one that responded to domestic and international emergencies, medical advancements, and the daily needs of the patients they served.

Throughout the first four decades of the twentieth century, recruitment standards for the ANC remained the same as McGee's requirements for nurses. Women had to pass a series of strict physical, moral, mental, and professional exams in order to gain admission to the nurse corps.[54] The exams excluded male nurses from the ANC ranks and made it difficult for African American women to qualify for the corps. Therefore, the ANC, like much of the U.S. nursing field, remained a white female institution. These standards and policies also resulted in continued personnel shortages during the ANC's most critical periods, World War I and World War II. Exceptions to these arrangements generally occurred at critical points during a conflict and challenged perceptions about the connection between race, sex, and nursing ability.

African American Women Nurses

For African American nurses, the introduction of formal nurse training during the last quarter of the nineteenth century did not result in a significant expansion of opportunity in the public sphere or the labor market. Instead, nurse training represented an enforcement of racial exclusionary policies that obstructed their access to the occupation. White nursing schools denied admission to African American women or restricted them to a small number in training schools well into the 1890s.[55] Furthermore, the growth of professional associations—meant to govern and shape the emergent profession—restricted membership only to those women who were alumni of recognized training schools or could take their state license exams, to which African Americans rarely gained access. This meant that African American nurses were denied both national and local recognition of their place within the growing profession.[56] As a result, African American nurses created their own professional organization to advocate on their behalf and combat discrimination.

The 1908 founding of the National Association of Colored Graduate Nurses (NACGN) established a support system for black nurses. Its mission throughout its forty-two-year history was threefold: improve professional standards for nursing, "develop leadership within the ranks of the NACGN," and challenge discrimination.[57] Challenging racial discrimination was especially important to the NACGN because discrimination formed the single largest barrier to African Americans in the nursing profession by keeping African American females out of most training programs and many hospital jobs. By extension, the NACGN argued, discrimination and its effects resulted in deficient healthcare for all Americans, including minorities.[58] To that end, members of the NACGN participated in a number of activities meant to reflect their abilities as nurses with the hopes of gaining recognition and unrestricted membership in national nursing groups such as the American Nurses' Association.[59] While largely unsuccessful, according to historian Darlene Clark Hine, their activities during the first two decades of the twentieth century reinforced both their desires and their dreams. They looked to the emerging war emergency as an opportunity to achieve their goals.[60] The attention of the NACGN shifted its focus to integrating the ANC as the country moved into World War I.

The use of African American nurses in the U.S. Army was not a new concept in the second decade of the twentieth century. African American nurses and black soldiers labored with the army in both the Civil War and the Spanish-American War. Yet their employment in the newly founded auxiliary to the Army Medical Department was atypical. Admission to the ANC occurred in coordination with the American Red Cross Reserve.[61] Black nurses did enroll in the Red Cross Reserve during World War I, but the Red Cross did not expect the army to employ them. Many Red Cross administrators believed black nurses' qualifications were inferior to those of white nurses and therefore relegated black nurses to the bottom of the pool of available nurses. In addition, the U.S. Army and Surgeon General were quick to note that there were no available or suitable quarters for black nurses.

A vocal campaign by the NACGN demanding that African American nurses be moved to the priority list of available nurses did little to change the status of nurses wishing to support their country. Instead, a medical emergency once again functioned as the linchpin that drew African American nurses into military service. The 1918 influenza crisis stretched both civilian and military medical services, and the army finally conceded the need for extra nurses and inducted eighteen African American nurses in the fall. They served in a segregated unit for a short time, just nine months.[62] Even so, as with black soldiers, race advocates saw in the military service of African American nurses the space to demand extended citizenship rights and independence from the strictures of racism. Black nurses understood their aspirations during World War I as part of a campaign for justice, and the wartime experiences of African Americans reinforced their determination to participate fully in both civilian life and as part of the military of the United States.[63] Yet the Great War of 1914–1918 proved once again that while war conditions may bend the strictures of social expectations—especially concerning gender roles and race relations—the end of the war resulted in a quick return to the status quo. Nevertheless, the lessons of the World War I experience left a legacy that race advocates built upon in the interwar period. The ANC reduced their numbers, but black nurses—restricted from both military participation and several national professional associations— doubled their efforts to achieve recognition and end discrimination.

Some eighty years after the Civil War, African American women and (and, later, white males) used wartime demands on the profession not only to gain recognition but also to challenge their own second-class status in the occupation. As we will see in the next chapter, the growth of civil rights organizations, including the expansion of NAACP branches throughout the United States during World War II and the expansion of a broader civil rights movement, signaled that African American men and women would no longer tolerate Jim Crow.[64] It also changed the way Americans understood rights and access to the benefits of citizenship. African Americans, in particular, used wartime rhetoric about equality and democracy on behalf of their campaign for equal rights, justice, and opportunity. At the same time, African American women employed traditional gender conventions as one of their strategies in their integration campaign. The consequences of this campaign, then, were successful and unsuccessful attempts to reorganize race and gender roles in American cultural understandings of place and occupation of its citizens and society.

2

"The Negro Nurse—A Citizen Fighting for Democracy"

African Americans and the Army Nurse Corps

> We the Wives, an Organization of Service Men's Wives, appeal to you in the name of our fighting husbands who are in desperate need of adequate medical care to utilize to the fullest extent the services of all nurses, regardless of color.
>
> —Telegram to the U.S. Armed Forces in a mass campaign to end race restrictions in nursing.

Even as the United States entered World War II to protect freedom and democracy, discrimination against its racial minorities continued as the nation's greatest dilemma. Rather than take the initiative to integrate the United States military, the War Department continued to privilege Jim Crow policies in the nation's fighting force. African American women, like the servicemen's wives quoted above, insisted that these policies harmed the cause to which the United States was dedicated.[1] The policies also harmed American soldiers by limiting the nurses accepted for service and by restricting where some nurses—particularly African American female nurses—served. By early 1945, perceived nursing shortages provoked the War Department to consider a draft of female nurses. Stunned by the possibility of drafting women, black and white citizens questioned the army's continued ban on the use of black female nurses when nurse leaders and media reports publicized their wide availability. African American female nurses used this moment to garner further support in their long-standing campaign to integrate the Army Nurse Corps. Public protest against drafting women into the military helped remove the final barriers against this integration. It was, however, a successful collaboration between African American nurses and race organizations and leaders, and the interracial connections cultivated by black nurse leaders during the exigencies of war, which ultimately forced the military to reevaluate their race policies.[2]

The campaign to integrate the Army Nurse Corps (ANC) reveals more about the acceleration and strengthening of a larger and wider civil rights movement than is commonly known to most Americans. Two decades before the passage of *Brown v. Board of Education* heralded in the "classical" phase of the civil rights movement, civil rights activists, as well as labor unionists, liberal New Dealers, and even black and white radicals, worked to overturn the race, class, and gender inequalities they saw as the hallmarks of the modern state.[3] These activists and those in the twenty years following World War II continuously challenged what historian Nancy MacLean termed the "culture of exclusion."[4] At the heart of this challenge was the struggle to gain "full and fair" access to the benefits of citizenship. Therefore, it was not just a question of overcoming racial discrimination. Rather, challenging a "culture of exclusion" simultaneously necessitated working to end economic discrimination and exploitation, while expanding social welfare policies that were characteristic of liberal New Dealers and labor unionists in the decade before World War II.[5]

In the early war years, concerns about race mixing along with outright racism influenced military nursing policies just as they had shaped similar policies for the rest of the U.S. Armed Forces. The army originally had no plans to employ nonwhite nurses.[6] Rather than have black nurses and white nurses work together, which was occurring increasingly and without incident in larger civilian urban hospitals, or having black nurses attend to white soldiers, the army rejected either course in the prewar years.[7] The War Department and the surgeon general reconsidered this stance only after protests from black nurses and race leaders, and then suggested a minimal use of black nurses after the U.S. Army accepted black soldiers. Increasing nurse shortages raised serious questions about the necessity of keeping race politics and policies in place. In order to attract more women into the occupation, recruitment campaigns touted nursing as "war work with a future" and emphasized the occupation as a natural extension of women's abilities with suitable pay.[8] Nevertheless, the military continued to restrict access to its two nurse corps almost entirely to whites.[9] The majority of African American female nurses were therefore racially excluded from taking advantage of the "work with a future" or performing the work assigned to their sex—according to recruitment campaigns. How could African American women or African Americans in general participate in, thrive in, and defend the nation under such conditions?

This question was the most important for those working to break down the barriers to black participation in the war effort. Black female nurses and their supporters implicitly recognized that integrating the ANC during World War II could not be an insular movement. They and civil rights advocates understood the struggle as part of the larger civil rights campaign for the full rights and benefits of citizenship. A 1942 nursing newsletter, for example, reminded black nurses of the importance of adhering to the Double V campaign of the *Pittsburgh Courier*. In this way, the integration of the nurse corps was connected to the national "victory at home, victory abroad" civil rights campaign.[10]

Nurse leader Estelle M. (Riddle) Osborne considered the significant role African American nurses played in a larger civil rights movement. In her view, nursing epitomized the complexities of race relations and discrimination. This occupation was widely assumed to provide care and comfort for those who are ill. Unfortunately, persistent cultural influences and racist practices unfairly regulated who provided care and how it was distributed. Four years after the end of World War II, Osborne recalled, "Professional relations in nursing [were] so interwoven with race relations that it has been imperative for Negro nurses to move on both fronts simultaneously to achieve their goals."[11] Osborne's casual reference to the position of African American nurses is perhaps the clearest expression of the monumental task faced by black nurses and, in fact, by the entire African American population. Nurses had to support the war effort in order to defend democracy, while simultaneously pushing for an end to discrimination and access to the full rights due to all U.S. citizens.

African American nurses in this quandary constantly struggled between searching for economic opportunity and professional recognition on one hand, and challenging discrimination and racism on the other. While the nursing profession struggled to professionalize, black nurses faced the additional burden of dealing with race prejudice.[12] They sought recognition from both the medical establishment and from the nursing profession. Even recognition, however, did not guarantee an end to discrimination. Black nurses, like black men, hoped that service to their country would result in full citizenship.[13] Thus, military service during World War II acquired special meaning to African American female nurses, especially after the failure to achieve civil rights goals after World War I. This time, they expected to be rewarded for their military service and to participate fully in both civilian and military life in the United States.

Black Nurses Organize

After the founding of the ANC as an auxiliary of the U.S. Army Medical Corps in 1901, Congress determined that the nurse corps would be composed solely of women.[14] This restriction was the result of both convention and politics. First, persistent cultural and societal beliefs characterized women as having a unique and natural temperament to care; on this basis, the nurse corps excluded men.[15] Further, as nursing scholars have noted, popular perceptions viewed nursing as a task based mostly on emotion and an altruistic ethic, consisting chiefly of menial work and linked to the domain of women, too demeaning for men.[16] Second, at the turn of the twentieth century, middle- and upper-class white women lobbied for the formation of a permanent ANC. Their goal was to create a respectable job for their daughters. These attitudes defined the organization's existence well into the mid-twentieth century.[17] Only through appointment by the surgeon general and the approval of the secretary of war did women achieve admission to the ANC. Extremely stringent guidelines and exams, as well as explicitly racist practices, limited the nurse corps primarily to educated white women.[18] Although both groups contested these guidelines, the early ranks of the ANC excluded minority female nurses and white male nurses. The few exceptions to these standards occurred in emergencies and never included male nurses. The first exception occurred during World War I.

Nursing shortages in 1918, created by war casualty rates and the influenza outbreak, allowed for the induction of eighteen African American nurses into the ANC. This exception, born of desperation, did not reverse the belief that black females were not suitable for the ANC: basic necessity forced the Red Cross and the army to call any reserve nurses registered with the Red Cross. Nearly two dozen women served at three army training bases: Camp Sherman in Chillicothe, Ohio; Camp Grant in Rockford, Illinois; and Camp Sevier in Greenville, South Carolina. Serving their country remained with these women despite their disillusionment over their temporary acceptance in the nurse corps. "The story of the Negro nurse in World War I is not spectacular. But each one of us . . . did contribute quietly and with dignity to the idea that justice demands professional equality for all qualified nurses," wrote Aileen Cole Stewart.[19] Out of this experience, black nurses began to challenge ANC policies and the discriminatory attitudes that permitted them no more than a temporary position in the military. For many black activists, the barriers black nurses faced in civilian nursing and in their quest for military service became symbolic of the professional and personal struggles of African Americans in general. Inspired by A. Phillip Randolph's linking of the Brotherhood of Sleeping Car Porters' unionization efforts at the Pullman Railroad Company to broader demands for black rights, black activists saw similar possibilities in the campaign of nurses during World War II.[20] Overcoming race discrimination and segregation in a vocation intimately tied to the health and well-being of American society would signal one more space wherein African Americans refused to accept the status quo.

Healthcare and access to medical services affected the lives of the black community. Already in 1915, Booker T. Washington had founded the National Negro Health Week Movement to increase health awareness and life expectancy among blacks, as racism and discrimination in the American medical establishment made access to healthcare and the training of black medical professionals difficult. By the 1930s, African American concern over civil rights involved healthcare as much as any other social, political, or economic issue. When addressing civil rights and healthcare matters, black community leaders and academics supported an increase in the number of available black health professionals and medical facilities.[21] Twice between 1937 and 1949, the *Journal of Negro Education*, for example, devoted entire issues to the health status and education of African Americans in the United States. The journal's contributors believed that the "health of the Negro is a matter of vital concern for the race and for the nation."[22] By connecting the healthcare of the nation with the health of its racial minorities, race activists strategically highlighted the interdependence of a healthy citizenry and the health and success of the nation. "Any group—white, black, or red—subjected to unhealthy environmental influences will present an unhealthy social picture," one black nursing leader reminded her audience.[23] In other words, a healthy nation needed healthy citizens, regardless of race, and that required African American access to acceptable medical training and healthcare programs.

Access to hospitals, training schools, and employment varied, however, and depended largely on the state and region where individuals lived. Even where training schools or employment opportunities existed for African Americans, recognition and opportunity—as in the case of black nurses, for example—did not always follow from that training.[24] Integrated hospitals that trained or employed African Americans were often located in the Northeast and Midwest, far from the large populations of African Americans living in the rural South in the mid-1930s.[25] Black leaders, therefore, understood well the direct impact of racism on the state of black healthcare. Census estimations from 1937 indicate that the African American population in the United States consisted of one-tenth, or twelve million people, of the general population, yet the number of black doctors and nurses were four thousand and six thousand, respectively. This meant that the ratio between black doctors and patients was about 1 to 3,000. Comparatively, the ratio of white doctors to the white population was 1 to 744.[26] The availability of black nurses was not much better, as most black nurses chose northern urban areas over southern rural regions that desperately needed them.[27] A combination of racism, economics, and hospital facilities presented African American female nurses with better wages and work opportunities in northern urban areas.

The lack of black nurses posed a special problem to the well-being of the black community. Nurses were often the first or only medical contact many rural blacks had. Yet during the 1920s and 1930s white nursing professionals showed little interest in improving the training of black nurses to raise the overall health status and care of African Americans. Certainly, educating more black nurses was part of a larger discussion about improving the nursing profession among national nursing groups such as the American Nurses' Association, the National Organization of Public Health Nurses, and the National League for Nursing Education. The American Nurses' Association organized a "Committee to Study the Status of Colored Nurses" in the late 1920s but did little to translate the committee's findings into expanded professional and educational opportunities for black nurses.[28] White nurses, according to scholar Patricia D'Antonio, "held the privilege of race" in that the advantage of race served white nurses.[29] The white-dominant nursing profession attempted to "eliminate weak nursing schools and to raise appreciably standards in remaining schools."[30] However, many of the schools they attempted to eliminate were the only training institutions accepting black nurses. These schools suffered less from a lack of standards than from a lack of financial and educational support. This only exacerbated racist presumptions that defined professional nurses as white and female. Poorly funded and largely ignored by most mainstream nursing associations, training schools for black nurses were widely viewed by whites as inferior, their graduates as less competent.[31] These presumptions undermined the ability of African American female nurses to provide care for patients and translated into low status and negative attitudes against black nurses inside and outside the nursing field.

By the 1930s perceptions about the importance of nursing to the medical and healthcare of patients had shifted. The progressive impulse of the first few decades of the twentieth century incorporated a revision of nursing standards as part of a heightened awareness of communal social welfare. While technically categorized as a semi-profession—a title nursing leaders argued against—the African American community often bestowed and used the title of "professional" for nurses.[32] In fact, most Americans viewed nursing as an integral part of the welfare of communities; medical professionals, especially, understood that the availability of well-trained nurses greatly affected the community. Even while revisions in professional nursing standards appeared detrimental to the educational opportunities for African American female nurses, they proved invaluable to the black nurses who began working to revitalize a national black nursing association. For the black community, nursing emerged as an important arena to fight racism and discrimination. Race organizations considered caregiving as one area of common ground for all Americans. Although debates continued about how well certain members of American society could provide care, everyone could agree that better healthcare and more healthcare providers meant stronger, healthier individuals, and communities that were more productive. As one black nursing leader argued, "Too long the emphasis has been on racial differences. We need a New Deal in approach to community problems in order that we may recognize racial similarities."[33] Making racial cooperation and racial understanding in healthcare a national issue would benefit the entire nation.

The National Association of Colored Graduate Nurses (NACGN) provided a much-needed professional advocacy organization for all black nurses— private duty, public health, and hospital staff nurses.[34] Since its founding in 1908, however, the organization had suffered from a lack of membership, leadership, and financial support. The nurses found it difficult to pay monthly dues out of their already low wages. Some African American nurses, like their white counterparts, also saw no advantage in belonging to a professional association. Furthermore, the NACGN lacked any major benefactors to help with maintenance costs, and they had no office space to house the organization. Thus, the NACGN faced an uncertain future in its struggle to end racial discrimination and to aid in black nurse professionalization. The "convergence of three elements," according to one historian, led to its revival in the mid-1930s. These elements were the advocacy of key white nursing leaders and groups, the financial backing of white philanthropists, and new leadership of the organization.[35]

In a pivotal moment for nursing race relations, the National Organization for Public Health Nursing (NOPHN) conducted a survey focused on the disparities between white and black public health nurses in the early 1930s. The survey found blatant job discrimination, salary inequities, and an obvious lack of educational opportunity for black public health nurses as the

issues that hindered the group's success. It encouraged improved race relations among nurses as a means of strengthening and preserving professional
nursing autonomy.[36] The NOPHN recognized the importance of a united
nursing profession and hoped that the survey results would encourage the
American Nurses' Association (ANA) to ally themselves with black nurses.
They feared that the continued exclusion of black nurses from nursing dia-
logues and from the national nursing associations would force black nurses
to align with black doctors, not with other nurses. The American Nurses'
Association's Committee on Joint Relations reported: "There is special need
of the assistance of the American Nurses' Association at this time . . . since
the National Medical Association [the professional association of negro phy-
sicians] admits nurses and pharmacists, and has requested a joint committee
with the NACGN. These activities may tend to submerge the interests of professional nursing and retard the growth and advancement of the NACGN."[37]
As to the interests of professional nursing, the joint committee's comments
also highlight the fear that an alliance between the NACGN and the National
Medical Association might ultimately weaken hard-won nursing autonomy.
While neither the NOPHN's survey nor the Committee on Joint Relations'
report resulted in the acceptance of black nurses by the ANA, these documents increased the profession's awareness to the plight of black nurses. In the
mid-1930s, this, coupled with appeals for financial assistance by the NACGN,
led to generous financial patronage by Congresswoman Frances P. Bolton
of Ohio and the Julius Rosenwald Fund. The funds allowed the association
and its president-elect Estelle Massey Riddle to provide a salary for the first
executive secretary, Mabel K. Staupers, and to rent space for its headquarters
in the same building as several national nursing organizations, and not far
from the NAACP in New York City.[38]

The election of Riddle and hiring of Staupers proved advantageous for
the professional future of black nurses and the position of the nurses in
the political fight against discrimination and racism. Riddle and Staupers
brought extensive experience to the NACGN. Their wealth of administrative
knowledge and a history of working with white nurses helped them to build
coalitions among various healthcare groups that sought to advance the professionalization of nurses. Beyond the goals they shared with white female
nurses, Riddle and Staupers were also focused on civil rights activism. They
urged nurses to participate in "all racial-advancement work," encouraging
black nurses to forge relationships with local churches, schools, and other
black professionals, thus guaranteeing not only a continuous exchange of
information concerning the black community but also a wide dissemination

of information about black nurses, tying their plight into a larger civil rights matrix. Riddle and Staupers both demonstrated their dedication to racial advancement in their commitments beyond the NACGN. Riddle served as the second president of the newly formed National Council of Negro Women in 1935. Staupers cultivated relationships with the NAACP, the National Urban League, and members of the black press to strengthen the bonds between nurses and the communities they served.[39] These women differed, however, in their personal and working styles, which provided a well-balanced and multifocal approach to the association's goal of professional integration and civil rights activism.

Riddle, arguably the best-educated black nurse of her time, was a striking woman whose elegant, regal presence facilitated a comfortable working relationship with white nurses and philanthropists.[40] Born in Palestine, Texas, on April 3, 1903, she entered the Homer G. Philips Hospital Nursing School in St. Louis, Missouri, in 1920.[41] She graduated three years later, impressing the Missouri State Board Examiners with exceptionally high scores on her nursing exams.[42] Following graduation, she became the first black nurse to breech the "administrative color barrier," when she was appointed as head nurse of one of the wards in the hospital.[43] Riddle furthered her education at the Teachers' College at Columbia University, where she earned a bachelor of science degree in nursing and a year later became the first black nurse in the United States to earn a master of arts in nursing education. She became an instructor at the Harlem Hospital School of Nursing and the educational director of Freedman's Hospital in Washington, D.C. She returned to St. Louis and her alma mater to serve as its first black superintendent in the mid-1930s. Then, in the spring of 1934, she became president-elect of the NACGN.[44]

Staupers, in contrast, was outspoken, energetic, and, according to historian Darlene Clark Hine, played the "more visible role of 'interpreting the Negro nurse' to the general [white] public and marshaling mass support" on their behalf.[45] In this role, Staupers spent a great deal of time getting nurses interested in the association, speaking about the need for professional integration, and investigating the working conditions of African American nurses throughout the country. By the middle of World War II, Staupers was regularly corresponding and meeting with leaders of national race advocacy groups, white nursing leaders, military officials, and even First Lady Eleanor Roosevelt.

Born on February 27, 1890, in Barbados, Staupers moved to New York with her family in 1903 and entered the Freedman's Hospital School of Nursing in Washington, D.C., in 1914. After receiving her degree, she returned to New

York as a private-duty nurse. She helped organize the Booker T. Washington Sanatorium, serving as the institution's administrator and director of nursing.[46] Seeking to broaden her professional and administrative knowledge, Staupers briefly moved to Philadelphia, Pennsylvania. Exposed to segregation and to discrimination by staff and patients in Philadelphia, she aimed her activism, after this experience, at gaining full and equal opportunity for black nurses in the nation's healthcare system and among its professional nursing organizations. Throughout the 1920s and early 1930s she assessed and improved the healthcare of African Americans in Harlem and New York City.[47] Her appointment to the NACGN broadened her work to the national level.

Riddle and Staupers visualized a new direction for the association in the mid-1930s. They would place racism in the medical field at the forefront of discussions about democracy and the healthcare system in the United States. To do so, they sought the most extensive discussion of discrimination and racism. Their strategy continued the group's regional conferences that had begun with the first regional meeting of black nurses and their supporters at the Lincoln School for Nurses in New York in January 1934. By 1937 the NACGN had established four regions: Northeastern, Southeastern, West Central, and Southern. They also organized conferences at Hampton, Virginia; Louisville, Kentucky; Richmond, Virginia; and Nashville, Tennessee.[48]

The association envisioned these regional conferences serving three purposes. First, they provided an arena in which to discuss the status and problems black nurses and patients faced and then to set an agenda to attack those problems. Regional conferences allowed attendees to confront the most pressing problems near their origins, in local communities and at the state level. In the tradition of grassroots black activism, these conferences fostered lasting relationships with members of the communities they served; these relationships also bolstered the important status of nurses within the black community. As community leaders, their concerns therefore went beyond healthcare to the day-to-day struggles they and their patients faced. They were able to bring these concerns and problems to regional conversations and, through them, national conversations on the issues that most concerned African Americans.

Second, these conferences brought together key representatives of the national health leadership such as Mary Beard of the National Red Cross, Congresswoman Frances P. Bolton, the American Nurses' Association, the National Organization for Public Health Nursing, and the National Health Circle for Colored People. The gathering of these leaders and organizations emphasized the importance of increasing interracial cooperation and interaction. The NAACP echoed this sentiment. Riddle and Staupers understood that this was vital to further their cause. According to Staupers, interracial cooperation challenged "community patterns that . . . hindered free communication between Negro and white nurses, and between the Negro nurses and concerned citizens."[49] White support, especially from prominent citizens such as Congresswoman Bolton and Eleanor Roosevelt, publicized and legitimized the black nurses' campaign. It also paved the way for those who might be uncomfortable or unwilling to work with African Americans.

Finally, these conferences brought together nurses and representatives from civil rights organizations.[50] Walter White of the NAACP, for example, regularly corresponded with the leadership of the NACGN. A year after the start of World War II he agreed to meet with Judge William Hastie (the African American lawyer, former judge, and civilian aide to the Secretary of War) and Mabel K. Staupers on the "matter of integrating Negro nurses into the Army Nurse Corps."[51] He also exchanged political strategies and discussed a variety of race issues with Staupers and Riddle.[52] Staupers and White exchanged letters on continuing discrimination on railroads, for example, and Staupers was later invited to represent the NACGN at a national political-strategy conference attended by race leaders to discuss the 1944 presidential election. Riddle reminded nurses of the importance of such relationships. She wanted nurses to concern themselves not only with nursing but also with "changing social and economic conditions," matters which also affected the future of nursing and nurses.[53] The NACGN also emphasized the commonality of purpose among all black organizations. In their August 1942 *News Bulletin*, nurses were told, "We are urging all local and state associations to cooperate with the Double-V for Victory campaign of the *Pittsburgh Courier*. Besides working for Democracy abroad, we must work for Democracy at home. Nurses too well know what it means to be denied Democracy."[54] Again, the relationship with national race organizations allowed female nurses to see their campaign as a contributor in the growing civil rights movement. In this way, Riddle and Staupers differed from their predecessors; they envisioned nurses and their activities as playing an important role in strengthening the black rights movement.

Wartime Healthcare and Home-Front Racial Politics

Segregation and discrimination in the military grabbed the interest of civil rights organizations well before the United States entered the hostilities of World War II. As concerns about the numbers of nurses became the focus of military and home-front preparedness, black nurses seized the attention of national white nursing leaders. During the interwar period, African American female nurses, mainly through the NACGN, had sought, in vain, for inclusion in the armed forces nurses' corps and in the national discussions about healthcare.[55] During the 1930s black nurses found some validation for their organizing efforts. Nevertheless, as nursing leaders acknowledged the importance of black nurses in mobilization efforts, racial politics simultaneously restricted their role.

In late September 1940 the White House convened a conference to discuss the National Defense Program. The list of invitees included members of the NAACP and the NACGN, signaling that the president recognized a role for African Americans in the upcoming war. About the same time, nursing leaders from around the country founded the Nursing Council for National Defense and hosted a conference to discuss wartime national healthcare. As members of the Nursing Council, the NACGN participated in the conference. At both events, discussions included providing Negro nurses with the full opportunity to serve "in the Army, the Navy, and the Red Cross."[56] Optimistically, for nurses and race leaders, these conferences offered a sense that their hard work had paid off. They concluded that healthcare leaders, along with the military, defense, and governmental agencies, finally recognized the need to employ *all nurses* in the care of American people, especially those in the Armed Forces.[57] African American nurses expected that changes in ANC policies would ensure the full employment of black nurses in the wartime organizing: after all, President Roosevelt informed Walter White of the NAACP that impending announcements would "insure that Negroes are given fair treatment on a non-discriminatory basis."[58] Moreover, Roosevelt's assurances of "fair treatment" made the goal of ending racism and discrimination in the country seem much closer.[59]

The NACGN mobilized its own Special Defense Committee as a cautionary measure to support the nurses further. From experience, the NACGN, especially Executive Secretary Staupers, did not trust that black nurses would be allowed to serve their country, regardless of the announcements to that effect. The Special Defense Committee guaranteed that the voice and problems of black nurses were presented to the white-dominated wartime healthcare committees. The Special Defense Committee kept the NACGN leadership apprised of developments concerning black nurses, but they were also a vital visual representation of all black nurses, reminding whites of their existence and determination. The shrewd planning of the NACGN paid off. The committee's existence was fortunate because African American leaders faced contradictory messages from the War Department and President Roosevelt in 1940 and 1941.[60]

In October 1940 members of the NACGN Special Defense Committee met with Julia O. Flikke, the chief of the ANC, and James C. Magee, the surgeon general of the United States Army, to discuss the release of the War Department's "plan for the use of colored personnel." Drafted by the Office of the Surgeon General and the War Department, the plan stipulated that no "'colored personnel' would be called into service until separate black wards would be designated . . . and only where the number of black troops warranted separate facilities." Members of the Special Defense Committee were disappointed. This plan clearly contradicted the president's statement that indicated fair treatment and opportunity to African Americans in wartime preparation. In response, Magee and Undersecretary of War Robert F. Patterson noted that the plan was "entirely consistent with racial policies and customs operating in the larger society," and in a nod to the Jim Crow mentality of the period, they declared that segregation was not discrimination because it afforded equal facilities to African Americans.[61] These comments invigorated the Special Defense Committee, which quickly informed the surgeon general that they would "sustain an organized protest to their Representatives in Congress." Magee's and Patterson's attitudes also strengthened the resolve of civil rights advocates regarding civilian and military integration. The activists used Magee's and Patterson's comments to challenge the continued application of the "separate but equal" doctrine that perpetuated a racist status quo among American citizens.[62]

Before 1941 African Americans did not ignore the military's call for nurses. Hoping to participate, black nurses rushed to the nearest Red Cross recruitment location to join the nurse corps.[63] The vast majority, however, faced outright rejection during the first few years of the war and a less-than-welcoming acceptance during the final years of the war. From one black nurse, Staupers learned: "In reply to your letter of Sept. 27, 1940, I regret to tell you that your application for appointment in the Army Nurse Corps cannot be given favorable consideration as there are no provisions in Army Regulations for the appointment of colored nurses in the Nurse Corps. . . . It is regretted that circumstances preclude a more favorable reply."[64] After receiving several similar letters from disheartened black nurses, Staupers pleaded with the president to "do something to remove this stigma from the Negro nurse." Staupers, like A. Philip Randolph, hoped that her direct appeal to Roosevelt about the role of African Americans in the war might pressure him to take decisive action against the blatant discrimination. Further, Staupers also let the president know that the fight to secure the full admission of black nurses into the ANC would not go away: "We have prepared ourselves . . . and can see no reason why we should be denied service in the Army Nurse Corps."[65]

Less than a week after Staupers wrote to the president, the surgeon general's office notified Staupers of two important decisions. First, the use of "colored nurses in the Medical Department of the Army as reserve nurses" was under consideration in the War Department. This meant that the War Department at least recognized that there would be a need for black nurses.[66] Second, together with the release of the War Department's "plan for use of colored personnel," the surgeon general and Medical Department of the army proposed the use of a small number of African American female nurses to care solely for black soldiers in locations dominated by segregated troops. In this way, General George C. Marshall believed the War Department was protecting "the social relationship between negroes and whites which has been established by the American people through custom and habit."[67] The army could avoid, or at least lessen, any fears or protest about race mixing in its medical department; black nurses would be concerned primarily with nursing black American soldiers, leaving white nurses to care for white soldiers. The military had no intention, Surgeon General Magee later declared, of allowing "colored nurses or colored physicians" to "be engaged in the care and treatment of military personnel other than colored."[68] If this was not enough to drive home the command's belief about "race mixing," the inferiority of African Americans, and the limited use of blacks in the war effort, General Marshall also noted that "either through lack of educational opportunities or other causes the level of intelligence and occupational skill of the Negro population is considerably below that of the white."[69] Yet the decision by the War and Medical Departments and the new policy concerning the use of black nurses brought up some troubling issues for nurses and civil rights activists; the army implemented segregated medical care for soldiers and the segregated stationing of black nurses where no historic precedent existed.

Following a meeting in March 1941 that included the National Defense Committee of the NACGN, Surgeon General Magee, and Judge William Hastie, the NACGN issued a statement on the "Status of the Negro Nurse in the Army Nursing Corps." The association pointed to the earlier precedent concerning race relations in the ANC. During World War I, black nurses served in an integrated army for their few months of service; they attended both black and white soldiers at Camp Sherman and Camp Grant, and they worked alongside white nurses with little complaint. In addition, black and white nurses were working together in civilian hospitals in cities such as "New York, Los Angeles, Cleveland, Chicago, and Boston"; indeed, at one eastern hospital operated by blacks, whites made up a large minority of their patients. Black nurses and activists wanted to know what was different now. Why was the surgeon general so intent on taking segregation to such extremes during the current conflict? The answer may be found in the increasing integration in many larger hospitals in the country and fears about how that might translate into other areas of the civilian society.[70]

During peacetime, the army admitted that arranging separate quarters and dining facilities made it impractical to appoint black nurses to the nurses corps, especially with so few permanent black regiments, but the World War I experience demonstrated it was not impossible.[71] According to one 1927 letter, "white and colored soldiers are not segregated in military hospitals," so while this meant the addition of black nurses was not necessary, it also meant that white nurses attended both races.[72] Additionally, the letter claimed that that army believed that black nurses performed satisfactorily during World War I. Herein lay one point of contention between Surgeon General Magee's decisions and activists' responses to them. The country was not yet at war in 1940 and 1941. For the surgeon general and others, the admission of a few dozen black nurses out of extreme necessity—as was the case during World War I—was quite different from their full acceptance into the ANC. His policies suggested an advantage to ignoring African American nurses until necessary or setting a limit on the number of black nurses needed to care for black soldiers.

In much the same way that the Red Cross vehemently continued to segregate blood and blood plasma, Magee believed he followed the opinion of the majority of Americans, even if these opinions were antithetical to war aims.[73] Therefore, the surgeon general refused to place "white soldiers in the position where they would have to accept [the] service of Negro professionals" or to have white professionals tend black soldiers.[74] In other words, if interracial care was happening in some civilian hospitals as the NACGN and NAACP claimed, it only occurred on a voluntary basis and in certain regions of the country. Many, including Senator Theodore Bilbo of Mississippi, praised the army and Magee for standing firm against attempts to use the military and the war to change existing social and racial hierarchies.[75] In contrast, African American nurses saw Magee's position as another example of keeping black American citizens from exercising their right to support their country and participate in the war. In response, the NACGN called on the NAACP, the black press, white nursing organizations, Congresswoman Frances P. Bolton, and the American Red Cross to support the full inclusion of black nurses.[76] Nevertheless, by early 1942 the allotment for black nurses in the War Department and the army remained small, with the inclusion of just sixty-five African American nurses.

In mid-1941, inconsistencies over the role of African Americans in the war effort grew more apparent, when President Franklin Roosevelt signed Executive 8802, which declared, "The policy of the United States [is] to encourage full participation in the national defense program by all citizens of the United States, regardless of race, creed, color or national origin, in the firm belief that the democratic way of life within the Nation can be defended successfully only with the help and support of all groups within its borders."[77] On the surface this was a major victory for African Americans. Indeed, this rhetoric, combined with notification from the Red Cross that the army welcomed all qualified black nurses, seemed to suggest that all Americans would participate in national defense. However, this also confused African Americans nurses. After originally indicating no plans to employ African American nurses, the War Department's plans then stipulated a severely restricted use of African American nurses in the defense of the United States in 1941.[78] While Roosevelt's executive order provided hope for black nurses, few changes occurred before 1943.[79] The black press kept African Americans acutely aware that Jim Crow was alive and well in the United States military with headlines that read "Appeal for Integration Is Ignored" and "Army Edict Bars Nurses: Need 30,000 but Decree White Only."[80] Quotas or allotments continued to restrict the number of African American nurses in the ANC. African American nurses served in the ANC only under the strictest of quota systems and only at bases where black troops either dominated or existed in a large enough number to require black nurses. Figure 1, a map illustrating the areas of division within the Army Corps and published in the December 1940 issue of the *American Journal of Nursing*, shows the placement of segregated bases in the United States and thus the locations of African American female nurses through 1943—primarily at Areas IV and VIII. By early 1944 fewer than 250 African American nurses were serving in the army. However, according to nursing census data and the NACGN, there were nearly eight thousand black registered graduate nurses in the nation. This meant that only about 3 percent of all African American nurses served in the army.

The existence of quotas was a recurring point of contention and source of confusion between black nurses and civil rights activists and the army and the War Department throughout the war. The quota system for African American nurses emerged early in war planning and was based on the number of black troops at segregated bases. For example, the War Department and Surgeon General Magee proposed a quota or allotment of fifty-six black nurses to serve African American soldiers in late 1940; Army Nurse Corps

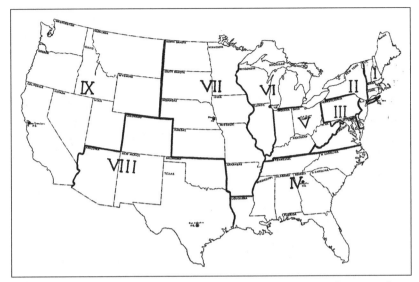

Figure 1. The map of the Army Corps Areas from 1940 illustrates the placement of segregated bases in the United States and thus the locations of African American female nurses through 1943. Black nurses were stationed mainly at bases in areas IV and VIII.

chief Julia Flikke suggested increasing the quota by as many as fifty more nurses just days after Pearl Harbor.[81] The use of quotas during World War II neither attempted to guarantee the acceptance of black nurses nor sought to integrate the military and open new opportunities to black nurses; rather, quotas limited the inclusion of African Americans in the war effort and in the armed forces of the United States. The War Department and the army decided where black nurses served and whom they cared for. By doing so, the army boldly asserted the second-class citizenship of black Americans while fighting a war ostensibly for democracy and equality.

During the first two years of the war, quotas guided the army's response to African American interest in joining the ANC. Black nurses received notification that the nurse corps either had reached its quota or was not currently taking applications from African American female nurses. Still, by late 1943 and early 1944, as the quota system supported a persistent nursing shortage, Surgeon General Kirk (mis)stated that there had never been a quota system. In response to Representative Robert Crosser, Kirk argued that the army never practiced discrimination in the acceptance and assignment of black nurses. Even though the army used the term "quota" consistently in correspondence with black nurses, Kirk stated, "there is not a quota system as applied to Negro nurses, unless it could be so regarded because of their assignment to specific hospitals." Instead, he argued that the "overall Army plans for allocation of troops," which designated the station assignments for the nurses, determined the number of African Americans nurses with the nurse corps.[82]

Ultimately, civil rights activists argued that the limited acceptance of black nurses into the ANC actually masked a scheme on the part of the army and War Department to exclude the service of most black nurses and to control the number and location of of black nurses they did employ. This mechanism maintained racial divisions; even more so, this policy, similar to those that assigned black soldiers to mainly noncombat positions, was yet another means of accommodating regional racial standards. Surgeon General Magee and Undersecretary of War Patterson openly acknowledged this fact early in the war. Supporters of black nurses as well as civil rights activists used this information to their advantage as the war progressed and nursing shortages became critical.

Black nurses embarked on a slow and painstaking course of action to push for integration. Staupers and other members of the NACGN began a brutal schedule of traveling the country to rally support for the nurse cause, to encourage black nurses to register with the Red Cross, and to investigate the lives of nurses in civilian and military environments. Their labor did help persuade some nurses to reapply for the ANC despite previous failures. One such nurse, Carolyn Dillon of New York, applied for the ANC. However, Dillon experienced a common result. The ANC replied to her application, "Your application for enrollment in the Army Nurse Corps cannot be given favorable consideration at this time because the quota of colored nurses required by the Corps has been filled . . . ; colored nurses are authorized for assignment only to those stations where colored troops predominate."[83] In light of numerous calls for nurses to support the war effort and join the ANC, such letters discouraged many nurses from applying. Frustrated, journalist Ruth Murray pointed out that the army and navy alike continued to stick to the "color line" even though both organizations only recruited half of the nurses they needed in September 1943. How could African Americans help the war effort when so few were wanted? Murray reiterated the warning issued by the chairperson of the interracial Joint Committee of Nurses: "The present discriminatory policy gives comfort to the enemy and is a gamble with the lives of fighting men."[84] How could black nurses defend democracy and equality when quotas and duty assignments for those nurses taken into the ANC did not reflect this ideal?[85]

Jim Crow influence on the war effort was a recurring theme in black newspapers and in the correspondence of leaders such as Staupers and Walter White. These black leaders marveled at "how America can say to the world that in this country we are ready to defend democracy when its Army and Navy is committed to a policy of discrimination."[86] In a series of articles in the *Chicago Defender*, African American writers named the army's continued support of Jim Crow policies as the root of low morale among the army's black military personnel.[87] "The morale of the Negro was drifting to low ebb because the government continued to allow anti-Negro agencies to hold the whip hand, and because of the abuse by the Army and the closed door policy of the Navy." These writers blamed the nursing shortage on the racist attitudes of a succession of men occupying the post of Army Surgeon General who believed that the army's practices toward black Americans did not amount to discrimination.[88] By late 1943 the national publicity garnered from these articles and an increasing shortage of nurses led to a turning point for African American female nurses. The nurses also gained support from the introduction of a national Cadet Nurse Program and a valuable ally to their cause in the form of the National Nursing Council for War Service. All helped to force the army and the nation to take the cause of African American nurses more seriously.

According to the U.S. Public Health Service, the "recruitment and training of enough nurses to meet both military and civilian needs" presented a most "serious and troublesome problem" for a nation at war.[89] By 1943, the competition from the lucrative opportunities for women in industry left nursing in an untenable position because women had to pay to be educated first. After lengthy discussions among nursing leaders about how to address this problem, Congress passed the Nurse Training Act of 1943, which established a federally subsidized nurse-training program known as the Cadet Nurse Corps. The federal program, Public Law 74, paid the tuition of women attending nursing school, provided a small monthly stipend, and offered living facilities with the expectation of increasing the number of nurses to meet military and civilian needs.[90] As the recruitment of women into wartime jobs advanced the idea of freeing up men to fight, the Cadet Nurse Program would use student nurses in hospitals as a way to free up graduate or trained nurses for military service. The cadet nurses would allow some nurses to enter military service, particularly nurses who were otherwise listed as essential personnel in hospitals and therefore not allowed to serve. Unlike previous attempts at increasing recruitment and training of nurses, the Cadet Nurse Corps proved beneficial even to African American women.

One of the main provisions of the Nurse Training Act was an antidiscrimination policy. The act "provided that the program for wartime education of nurses should be open to all, regardless of race, color, or creed." The passage of such an act revealed how critically low the numbers of available nurses had become by 1943. An advisory committee, consisting of nurses from around the country, including Estelle Riddle, helped determine which nurse-training programs met the regulations laid out in the Nurse Training Act. Schools interested in receiving access to federal aid benefited from opening their enrollment or collaborating with programs that trained both black and white nurses, and African American female nurses benefited from the vastly expanded educational opportunities. In the first two years of existence, the Cadet Nurse Corps saw nearly three thousand black nurses take advantage of the program. In a 1945 survey on black nursing, Riddle noted "a 21 percent increase in Negro students in the same number of schools over 1942" and an overall increase in "the number of schools admitting Negroes into mixed student enrollment." In 1943 the state of California alone reported that ten additional schools admitted black students along with whites following the 1943 commencement of the Cadet Nurse Corps program.[91] The Cadet Nurse Corps program, therefore, gave tangible incentives for the integration of nursing schools, and black nurses gained from expanded opportunity.

The Nursing Council for National Defense, a national clearinghouse for nursing organizations, discussed the role of nursing on the eve of World War II. The organization billed itself as the voice of nursing in Washington, D.C. when the discussion included wartime care. In 1942 the group changed its name to the National Nursing Council for War Service (NNCWS), broadening its membership to include not only "nursing organizations, but also hospital, medical, and both white and colored lay groups."[92] From its inception, the NNCWS facilitated interracial cooperation among black and white nurse leaders, at least in the form of including black nurses in the organization and in conversations about the war effort. By 1943, however, civilian and military needs heightened the National Nursing Council's concerns about black nurse discrimination and integration.

The NNCWS's focus on black nurse discrimination was an important move for the future of professional black nursing in civilian and military life. Along with the new Cadet Nurse Corps program, the support of the NNCWS meant that the black nursing cause became considerably broader in its focus. In February 1943, the council sponsored a meeting, "The Negro Nurse and the War." Leaders from nursing organizations, members of civilian and defense committees, directors of several nursing schools, and leaders from the NAACP and the National Urban League attended. A roundtable discussion, titled "The Negro Nurse—A Citizen Fighting for Democracy," focused on how to improve the employment and education opportunities and raise the recruitment of African American nurses. In this roundtable, participants acknowledged the particularly difficult and unique dual position held by a black nurse: "She is a member of a minority group fighting for its rightful place, and also a member of a profession still struggling for its proper place in the community." For this reason, the attendees agreed, the campaign to end discrimination against black nurses was especially important for both civilian and military nursing.[93] The NNCWS's strategy with this meeting was to publicize information about black nurses in order to quantify the effect of continued nurse discrimination on the lives of American fighting men. A 1945 report, "Facts about Negro Nurses and the War" for example, brought public attention to the "problems which troubled the Negro members of the nursing profession." The NNCWS worked closely with the NACGN, waging an all-out campaign to increase the number of nurses in the military and in civilian service. The NNCWS and NACGN argued that increasing the number of African American female nurses would add greatly to "military nursing resources" and would demonstrate the importance of American women, regardless of race, in the fight for democracy.[94]

The failure to employ all available nurses undermined the war effort. This becomes evident when comparing the number of men in the army with the total number of nurses in the ANC. By late 1944 there were eight million men in the army, of whom seven hundred thousand were African American. Yet of the nearly 44,000 Army nurses, only 330 were African American. This meant that for every white nurse, there were 166 white soldiers, but for every black nurse, there were 2,126 black soldiers.[95] This ratio was especially startling to activists who knew that most African American nurses remained in the United States and served only black troops or, in some cases, prisoners of war.[96] At the very least, the activists could argue, black soldiers serving abroad suffered from a lack of care. The comparison also revealed how continuing racism weakened the fight for democracy. At a ratio of one to nearly two hundred, white nurses, especially those close to combat areas, were overwhelmed, while black nurses stationed stateside found their services often underused. During the unique necessities of military conflict, segregation and discrimination's harm to both blacks and whites becomes dramatically undeniable.[97]

The report, prepared jointly by the NACGN and the NNCWS, highlighted race discrimination in the Nurse Corps and the serious nursing shortage.[98]

It found that "if as many Negro nurses—in proportion to their numbers—as white nurses were accepted by the Army" then "there would now be 1,520 Negro nurses in the Army . . . instead of the present 330."[99] At the heart of the report was the revelation—according to the NACGN and the NNCWS—that although many more black nurses were available and qualified for service, the army refused to increase their numbers in the Nurse Corps. The army's refusal to actively recruit and employ black female nurses where needed adversely affected the healthcare of the entire fighting force. The report concluded that it also reflected the poor use of manpower and continued discrimination against the nation's racial minorities. Nursing shortages—linked to race discrimination, according to black activists—would not disappear without an explicit policy by the military directing a change. Race leaders, such as Walter White of the NAACP, held some hope in 1944 that changes were on their way. The escalation of the war motivated some national and military leaders to construe improving race relations as a way to strengthen the war's mission of defending democracy.[100] These changes, however, were late and not nearly adequate to stem the nursing crisis.

The Nurse Shortage, a Nurse Draft, and Public Outcry

Most ANC records and public accounts suggest that while the number of nurses remained constant early in the war, by mid-1944 the supply had not kept up with the demand.[101] The demands for the recruitment of nurses fluctuated by as much as ten thousand from month to month in 1944. The U.S. Army recognized that as the perceived need for nurses increased, recruitment campaigns were not meeting the army's expectations. This situation was not due to a public that was unaware. According to the *American Journal of Nursing*, "78 percent of the population . . . were aware of the shortage of nurses" and were growing "increasingly impatient with the Army's refusal to use available nurses."[102] The *New York Times* noted that the army pushed to recruit one thousand nurses a month in the summer of 1944, while the surgeon general announced a month-long campaign to rally recruits for the Cadet Nurse Corps.[103] Still, the failure to remove the quotas on African American nurses bewildered most Americans who read about the estimated two thousand available black nurses in articles published across the nation in both white and black newspapers.[104] In the summer of 1944 the army considered a new strategy to recruit women who had nursing degrees but were not working as nurses.

In July 1944 the U.S. Army and War Department announced its decision to increase the number of black nurses serving with the nurse corps. Although the surgeon general maintained that no quota had ever existed in the army, both the white and black press labeled this step as the army's removal of racial quotas for the employment of nurses.[105] The *New York Times* reported that "nurses would be accepted without regard to race or creed," while a *Chicago Defender* headline read "Army Lifts Quota Ban on Nurses." Since the beginning of the war this was the first indication of any real breakdown of racial barriers. Nevertheless, the only assurances the surgeon general gave to those who questioned the assignment of African American nurses was to suggest that black and white nurses "will be assigned to positions they are best fitted to fill and where the maximum benefits can be secured from their services." In other words, the surgeon general offered no guarantee that the segregation of black nurses would cease with the acceptance of all qualified African American nurses.[106]

Indeed, while black newspapers heralded the apparent change in army policy as a long-awaited and hard-won victory for African American nurses, some members of the black press did not miss the opportunity to comment about the Army's complete turnaround with respect to the treatment of African Americans. They were skeptical and suspicious and, as the cartoon in Figure 2 suggests, warned not just black nurses but also the African American populace to be leery about the welcome. The ugly, masculine image of a white army nurse hides a "no negro nurse" sign behind her back, while aggressively pulling the highly feminized, attractive black nurse into the Army Nurse Corps. What did the complete acceptance of African American nurses really mean for African Americans? Clearly, the cartoonist worried about protecting African American females after their acceptance into a military organization and feared their loss of femininity and sexuality. The cartoonist hints that military nurses were unfeminine, asexual, or, even worse, "butch" and lesbian.[107] Further, although the army lifted its ban on the use of black nurses—represented by the chained dog in the cartoon—this did not mean that discrimination against African American nurses was at an end.[108] Superior officers' treatment of black nurses and duty assignment revealed that the admission of black nurses did not amount to equal treatment.[109] With few exceptions, African American nurses remained for the most part on segregated bases in the United States.[110]

Even after the July announcement, the chief of black nurses at the station hospital in a POW camp in Phoenix, Arizona, informed Staupers about the reality of black nurses' daily lives. In one letter, she discussed feelings of isolation both on and off the base. She informed Staupers, "We could not be served in any café or soda fountain," and while all white officers, including prisoners of war, had help cleaning their quarters, "we are the only women on

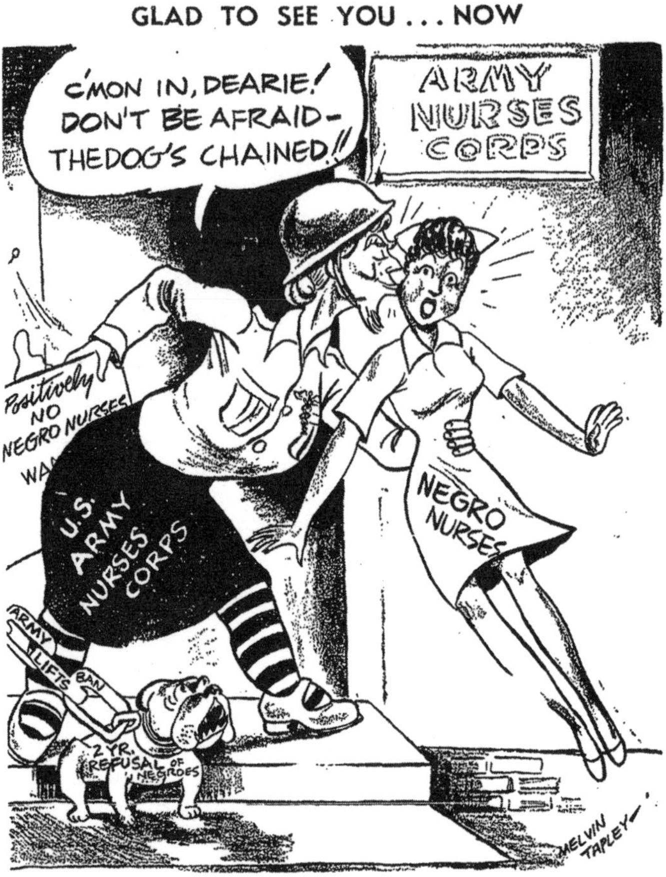

GLAD TO SEE YOU ... NOW

Figure 2. This cartoon was part of a series of cartoons created by Melvin Tapley that depicted racism and race relations in the United States during World War II. On military nurses, Tapley published two cartoons, commenting on the Army Nurse Corps and Navy Nurse Corps. Melvin Tapley, "Glad to see you . . . now!" *New York Amsterdam News*, July 22, 1944.

the entire post with no help whatsoever." She added further: "Apparently we are not considered officers by those in command for we are never included in the command affairs and meetings for all officers of the post to attend." Finally, she lamented, "As time goes by conditions seem to get worse than better." Ignored by command officers, refused service in town and on base, and treated with contempt even by prisoners of war, black nurses suffered the constant reminder of their place in military and civilian society. They were, apparently, little more than the tolerated help. Local citizens wanted the bases to provide everything that the nurses needed so they would not visit the local towns. The army's mismanagement of resources in assigning black nurses to too few locations in the United States compounded these unfavorable experiences. For instance, at Ft. Huachuca, there were 97 nurses caring for 110 patients at one point during the war.[111]

By August 1944, when casualty care in the war zones and for those returning to the United States peaked, officials in charge of nurse procurement realized they needed nearly sixty thousand nurses to meet demand. The Cadet Nurse Corps provided some relief, particularly in supplying civilian hospitals with student nurses, but the program was only a year old in mid-1944. Even with the cadet nurse program and the army's new policy concerning African American nurses, the ANC did not add black nurses proportionately. By mid-1944, just over three hundred African American nurses served in the army.[112] Regardless of the official end of restrictions against the use of African American female nurses, discrimination continued to block their participation. Officials continued to station black nurses on bases and in areas that catered mostly to black soldiers and prisoners of war. Even the small units of nurses deployed abroad spent a significant amount of time in some form of segregated settings either in housing, patient care, or duty assignment.[113] With little regard for the number of black female nurses available for appointment in the ANC, at the end of the year the surgeon general made the decision to send a number of general hospitals overseas without nurses.[114] While ANC records are unclear about the need for nurses with these general hospitals, the public was horrified to learn about the continuing nursing shortage and that hospital units were going overseas without nurses as a result. Such publicity advanced the idea of a female nurse draft among a larger public audience.

Quietly, conversations about drafting women, particularly female nurses, occurred for months within a larger conversation about Selective Service for all American citizens. In April 1944, a *Chicago Defender* article revealed that talk about a women's draft had elicited a government response. In a press memo dated March 30, 1944, the War Bureau of Public Relations declared: "Intimations that the Army was considering drafting nurses are incorrect. No such plans have been considered."[115] Despite this assurance, drafting female nurses became a viable option to deal with nursing shortages. In December 1944 journalist Walter Lippmann's scathing editorial pointed out that one cause of the nursing shortage was the fact that "women are not subject to the draft." He continued: "[O]nly an aroused and informed public opinion, focused as it may be by a Congressional inquiry, could break this logjam in the recruitment of women."[116] The draft was necessary, in his opinion, because American women, more concerned with comfortable, higher-paying civilian jobs, had failed in their obligation to the nation's fighting men. Lippmann's editorial, published in newspapers across the country, served as a call to arms to many in the public who were enraged by the apparent truth of Lippmann's claims. Unsubstantiated reports that suggested that soldiers were dying for want of care led some to see drafting nurses as the best means of addressing a desperate situation. Until Lippmann's editorial, few had spoken so publicly about the delicate subject of drafting women into military service. It was, after all, a radical idea; it would necessitate refashioning military service as an obligation and responsibility of not only American men but also American women. While this draft focused on a single group of women, some feared that, before long, all women would be subject to the draft.

Notwithstanding the concerns over drafting women, President Roosevelt was disturbed by reports that recruitment had failed and nursing shortages persisted. On January 6, 1945, the president announced to Congress his support for legislation to expand the Selective Service Act of 1940, which would include, for the first time in American history, the drafting of female nurses into the army.[117] The president's request to Congress was made more salient when Surgeon General Kirk declared: "It looks as if [the draft] will be necessary to meet the immediate need for nurses by a Congressional draft."[118] Three days later, Representative Andrew J. May's House Bill 1284, known as the Nurse Draft Bill, went to Congress and the Committee on Military Affairs. Roosevelt hoped that this bill would quickly resolve the nurse-shortage problem.

Roosevelt's proposal to Congress produced unpredicted results for both the president and supporters of the nurse draft. A public outcry quickly materialized in opposition to drafting female nurses.[119] Drawing upon the publicized availability of African American nurses, concerned citizens and supporters of black nurses went on the offensive. The proposed draft even sparked a confrontation between Staupers and Surgeon General Kirk. Lamenting the underutilization of qualified African American women, Staupers asked Kirk, "If nurses are needed so desperately, why isn't the Army using colored nurses?"[120] She then used her connections through the NACGN to rally opposition to the nurse draft. She pointed out the hypocrisy of "calling for a draft of nurses while excluding large numbers of black nurses willing to serve."[121] She asked supporters of African American female nurses to write to the White House, their congressional representatives, and the media to call attention to the availability of women for service.

Telegrams supporting the use of black female nurses inundated the White House from groups as varied as the NAACP, the American Federation of Labor, United Church Women, and the National Council of Negro Women. One urged, "Mothers and Fathers of America: It is your sons that may never return because of inadequate nursing . . . telegraph or write to your Senators and Representatives today."[122] Members of Congress received an abundance of these letters. Edith Nourse Rogers of Massachusetts received letters that chastised her support of the nurse draft and questioned the failure of employing African American women. "It is a deplorable situation. It means that the officials in charge of nursing services believe it is better for their service to go understaffed than to be staffed by negroes."[123] The acting secretary of the National Negro Congress wrote to the president that "the nation-wide support which [black nurses have] received on this specific issue, we believe, indicates that our nation and the armed forces generally are ready to accept Negro nurses on a basis of full integration."[124] The NACGN even released a statement concluding that any bill extending the Selective Service Act to women nurses should "be amended in order that the service to American soldiers be placed on the basis of need for nursing care and not on the basis of limitations because of race, creed, or national origin."[125] Black nurses and their supporters emphasized one important fact: women nurses willing to care for soldiers did exist, but race discrimination kept them from doing so.

Their campaign for full integration was strengthened because black nurses publicly exposed the flaws in the female draft bill and the public fear that American soldiers were dying because of nursing shortages. As one historian described it, "Roosevelt apparently had not the slightest appreciation for the depth of the public's dissatisfaction with the armed services' restrictive [policies] towards nurses."[126] Public opinion saw only one viable option: allowing black nurses to join the ANC was preferable to the drastic measure of drafting even a very small segment of the female population.

Just two weeks after President Roosevelt's radio address to Congress, the surgeon general and the War Department jointly declared an end to exclusionary racial practices. The ANC would now accept, without regard to race, all qualified nurses.[127] This was indeed a major success for African American female nurses and the NACGN. Only six months before, however, the army had made a similar announcement. The drastic difference in the joint proclamation by the surgeon general and the War Department was a large, awakened public opinion.

Congress continued to debate the feasibility of drafting female nurses throughout the late winter and early spring of 1945. Yet by this time opposition to the draft had gained support, and recruitment numbers had increased. Those adamantly opposed offered several counterarguments. First, some nurses contended that drafting nurses for military service was the wrong approach, as it singled out a small population of American women.[128] In this way, a draft would discriminate against both sex and occupation. Catherine Dempsey, the president of the American Association of Industrial Nurses, argued instead that it would be fairer and more sensible to institute a universal draft for all women.[129] Second, drafting female nurses did not address the problem of how a shortage had occurred in the first place. Instead, the draft proposal drew attention to the military's racial and gender bias, evident throughout the war, as it had refused to fully employ African American nurses and had disregarded the use of male nurses.[130] Finally, some argued that proposals to draft nurses inherently focused on drafting *white* female nurses. If drafting nurses remained a possibility, the military needed to address these concerns.

Public opinion of black nurses had also changed as the war ended. Within a month of the surgeon general's announcement, a national opinion poll reported that more than half of the white adults surveyed were amenable to care by black nurses.[131] In a March 1945 issue of the *Trained Nurse and Hospital Review*, Janet Geister wrote: "I've often wondered, as I read that 'men are dying for want of nursing care,' if these men would cavil over the color or texture of the hands that might save them?"[132] Geister's response was directed to the ongoing draft debates, but her insightful comments expose how the exigencies of war provided the space and opportunity to challenge—temporarily in some cases—race and gender relationships in the United States. During World War II, the African American female nurses' campaign to integrate the ANC was best exemplified in the struggles for nursing service and nursing care. African American female nurses and their supporters questioned racial boundaries and argued for an inclusive civil rights movement, while promoting and strengthening traditional understandings of gender roles. Their promotion of traditional gender roles helped their cause and provided a victory for racial civil rights. However, male nurses who, employing a similar strategy, argued for integration at the same moment failed to breach the same barriers.

3

Nurse or Soldier?

White Male Nurses and World War II

So that the man who stands ready to meet
his country's call, shall, in his hour of need,
have the best that nursing care can give.

—Edith Aynes, *American Journal
of Nursing*, May 1940

With these lines, Second Lieutenant Edith Aynes closed her article on army nursing with the intent of encouraging nurses to remember their obligations and responsibilities and of making a clear delineation between the roles of men and women, even before U.S. involvement in World War II. This delineation defined soldiering and nursing in gendered terms, using sex difference to assign individuals to each occupation. Gender conventions and their articulation in the civilian nursing profession during the mid-twentieth century supported this prescription regarding the types of jobs available to nurses. The traditional assumption that soldiers were men and nurses were women required the government and military forces to confront the desires of men to take on a nonconventional role.

The existence of registered male nurses who wished to enlist in the military complicated this demarcation. Army Nurse Corps (ANC) policy and federal law deemed women the only suitable individuals to carry the title of "nurse" within the United States military medical structure. To address the puzzle of employing male nurses, the military attempted to assign male nurse volunteers and draftees to medical departments, with the rank of private and the title of "medical technician" or "corpsmen."[1] These bureaucratic measures fostered an already negative perception of male nurses while sustaining traditional gender divisions between nurse and soldier. Just as nursing shortages had acutely revealed the harmful effects of race restrictions on nursing care, gender restrictions exacerbated these circumstances at the height of World War II. The efforts by male nurses to gain recognition amid critical nursing shortages that initiated the bill to draft female nurses in early 1945 further underlined the problem of limiting the ANC to women.

Gender restrictions in the ANC and attempts to challenge them are an unstudied part of the politics of gender from the early days of war mobilization through the postwar period. Scholars such as Maureen Honey and Leila Rupp have pointed out the general continuity in traditional gender roles despite the attempt of mobilization propaganda to entice women into the workplace.[2] The "typing" of jobs—based on sex or race—had long guided employers in their hiring practices and was fundamental to institutionalizing both social and economic inequality.[3] Fearing the breakdown of traditional gender roles, wartime propaganda was careful to construct women's move into the workplace and military as temporary, thereby protecting what was, at any other time, the domain of men. The nursing profession was not immune to parallel fears—among female nurses—of encroachment by men into a female domain or the loss of a traditionally female job to men. Traditional ideals about womanhood, fear about the loss of autonomy, and what some women viewed as the need to protect womanhood shaped a good deal of the difficulty involved in integrating male nurses more fully into the profession and military even while nursing shortages grew.

Race's preeminent function in shaping social roles and beliefs in American society faced difficulties during World War II. In a pathbreaking article, Evelyn Brooks Higginbotham persuasively argued that race has functioned as a "metalanguage" historically, shaping notions of gender and sexuality and even overriding social perceptions of biological sex.[4] Through an examination of nineteenth-century court cases involving racial discrimination, Higginbotham challenged the primacy of gender in shaping the destinies of African American women and showed how racial thinking altered perceptions of womanhood before and after the Civil War. The different circumstances of African American women and white male nurses during World War II demonstrates how, under certain historical conditions, gender could overcome racial difference in breaking down systems of occupational segregation in some cases and maintaining them in others.

Far more than any other group of underrepresented nurses, the struggle by male nurses for recognition and acceptance in the ANC revealed the complex nature of equality. In much the same way that African American female nurses characterized their struggle as a fight against racism and discrimination, white male nurses also used the language of discrimination to describe their challenge. In an unusual set of circumstances, race limitations and gender restrictions within the ANC placed these two groups of nurses in similar, shared conditions. Male nurses, however, lacked the organization and numbers of African American female nurses. White men, who traditionally wielded power and authority because of their race and sex, found that gender conventions acted as their single greatest barrier in nursing. Their entrance into military nursing required not only a change in ANC policy and a reversal of congressional law, but also a revised public understanding of masculinity and nursing.

Continued sex and race discrimination in nursing schools and a narrow public opinion of who should qualify as a nurse placed white males at the center of the challenge of male nurse integration. The problem of segregation and racism meant that white men had more opportunity and means of challenging the barriers to the profession than men of any other race. By the early twentieth century, white men were more than 80 percent of the male nurse population. Estimates from the American Nurses' Association indicated that there were just over eight thousand white male nurses in the United States at the height of World War II. Between two thousand and three thousand of these men were active nurses and available for military service. These men trained at sixty-eight coeducational and four male nursing institutions that existed in the United States by 1941.[5] Nursing records also reveal that there were only 127 African American male graduate nurses and nurse students at the same time.[6] This could be for a variety of reasons, but as scholar Christine Williams points out, the circumstance most likely stemmed from the fact that most nursing schools were stratified by both race and sex. The basic education needed for nursing school and an environment of discrimination made nursing schools virtually closed to black men.[7]

The history of black male nurses is difficult to trace. Records of the National Association of Colored Graduate Nurses make little or no reference to black male nurses. Even the NAACP, when asked in 1940 about nursing schools that accepted African American men, could only reply, "We regret that we have no information on this topic . . . [and] we do not know of any who do."[8] This history is also difficult to recover. The femininity associated with nursing, "compounded by racial inequality," placed black male nurses in a position that required them to distance themselves from the profession in order to assert their masculinity.[9] Furthermore, nursing's historic connection to intimate contact made black men particularly "vulnerable to its gender images," according to historian Patricia D'Antonio, and made black male contact with white bodies nearly impossible.[10] The silence of these men therefore, speaks volumes about the race and gendered nature of the nursing profession. As a result, the struggle for male nurse equality and integration in both civilian and military nursing is almost exclusively the story of white male nurses.

Male Nurses and National Nursing Associations

In the United States, women dominated the occupation of nursing almost exclusively from its infancy. Since schools of nursing that trained men were rare and often associated with mental hospitals, the public knew almost nothing about men in nursing. The newly organized professional associations all but ignored male nurses. In 1897, a group of nurses in North America formed the Nurses' Associated Alumnae of the United States and Canada. In 1911 the U.S. nurses renamed their organization the American Nurses' Association (ANA). As with most nurse training schools that developed following Reconstruction, professional associations like the ANA reflected the evolution of the profession during the late nineteenth century. Following many of the tenets touted by Florence Nightingale, the ANA promoted the profession as properly and naturally occupied by women.[11]

Membership requirements and the organization's bylaws barred male nurses early in the ANA's history and reflected a gendered perspective on caregiving.[12] For example, until 1930 members were not only required to be graduates of training schools and members of their state associations, but their training had to include "practical experience in caring for men, women, and children."[13] This phrasing meant that male nurses did not qualify for membership. While the curriculum for men and women in nursing schools shared a great deal in common, male nurses were excluded from training in the pediatric and obstetrics/gynecological fields. They received instead training in urology and psychiatry.[14] This meant that men had little to no contact with either women or children and led some women nurses to view the men nurses as less skilled or competent practitioners. In 1924 male nurse Kenneth T. Crummer lamented that "the man who nursed was often frowned upon as an imposter, not a nurse, but an attendant or orderly of limited training."[15] This attitude led to a belief that male nurses were unworthy of professional recognition: one observer noted that men who nursed had no "representation in [professional] associations." The failure of professional nurse associations to "recognize the same need and protection for the man nurse in our profession" was a failure of professional organizations to fulfill their obligations to support and protect all nurses, the observer concluded.[16] Even as male nurses trained at some of the same institutions as female nurses or under the same educational tenets, the inability to participate in professional associations underscored the assumption that men nurses' limited job prospects defined a role somewhere between a trained nurse and a nurse's assistant. The opposite proved true for African American female nurses. Until the second decade of the twentieth century, African American women had little problem joining the American Nurses' Association. Race played an indirect factor only in determining which female nurses had access to membership in the ANA. They could gain professional recognition in the ANA in multiple ways.

Early in the ANA's history, membership required the affiliation with alumnae, state, or local nursing associations; therefore, a number of African American female nurses could and did join the ranks of the ANA. In 1916, however, as part of the reorganization of the ANA, the association changed its membership rules to stipulate that members must hold membership in their state associations. This barred most African American women from the organization, especially those who lived and worked in states that refused them membership in the nurse associations.[17] In contrast, male nurses, who would otherwise qualify for membership because of their connection to state associations, had little recourse to challenge bylaw requirements that excluded men from the ANA. Male nurses had no representatives among the ANA leadership; nurse training was firmly set against male nurse education in obstetrics or gynecology, while the 1916 changes to the ANA's bylaws defined membership requirements through training in these subjects and membership in state nursing associations. Unwittingly or not, the American Nurses' Association relied on both gendered and racialized conventions in determining whom it recognized as nurses in the first several decades of the twentieth century. As a result, until the ANA again amended its bylaws, the professional organization excluded a sizable majority of African American female nurses and all male nurses.[18]

The *American Journal of Nursing* deliberated on the position of men nurses in the profession several times in the years before the American Nurses' Association changed its bylaws to include them. As the voice of national nursing news—particularly two of the three national nursing organizations and dozens of state nursing associations—the *American Journal of Nursing* was, arguably, the most important forum for disseminating information to and about professional and student nurses.[19] Here, male nurses and their supporters found a platform from which to argue for professional recognition and to call attention to their perception of mistreatment by the wider profession. In a 1924 letter to the editor, a nurse identified only as M.H.R. remarked, "One of

[the] wrongs still waiting our attention and action concerns the male nurses of our profession and the recognition and place to which they have a *right* in our nursing world and with the public."[20] The question of equal rights was not far from the minds of many American citizens in 1924, especially women. Only a year before, Alice Paul and the National Women's Party introduced the first Equal Rights Amendment (ERA) to Congress. Its central premise was equality of rights regardless of sex. Published in the same volume as M.H.R.'s letter, prominent nurse leader Lavinia L. Dock detailed her support of the ERA; citing its importance to the labor industry, she suggested that the ERA would guarantee "equal rights and opportunities for adult men and women without restriction or exclusion based on sex alone."[21] Dock's emphasis on the idea of equal rights in her letter to the editor focused not only on the inequities faced by women in the labor market—one for which she blamed custom and common law—but argued also that this inequity harmed both men and women and future labor conditions. Yet she did not refer to the unequal conditions faced by men in her own profession, which was, by custom and common practice, deemed the protected domain of women. M.H.R.'s emphatic demand that the profession "right this wrong," then, alludes to broader implications of disregarding male nurses in professional associations. While female nurses could and did understand the importance of equal rights among the sexes, especially for the economic future of the nursing occupation, they often ignored or missed how they enabled sex discrimination and the continued gendering of the profession. By perpetuating bias against male nurses, and by failing to recognize trained male nurses as their professional equals, the ANA and other national nursing associations failed in their obligations to promote and support professional nursing on behalf of all nurses.[22]

Proposed amendments to the bylaws of the ANA failed throughout the 1920s, but discussions about male nurses continued during the period.[23] In 1928, for example, Kenneth Crummer pointed out that male nurse education and the job opportunities for graduate male nurses had expanded faster in the previous ten years than at any point since the turn of the century.[24] Still, it was not until the late spring of 1930 that a proposed amendment to the membership bylaws came to a vote. Members voted at the biennial convention in Milwaukee to approve the following addition to its membership requirements: "The training for male nurses must include practical experience in caring for men, together with theoretical and practical instruction in medical, surgical and urological nursing."[25] It is important to note that this proposal was only an addition to existing membership requirements; it did not necessarily reflect an acceptance of equality between male and female nurses, but it did recognize that male nurses needed access to professional representation. Tacked on to existing membership language, it removed the constraints keeping male nurses from the organization but did not attempt to write a single inclusive membership bylaw. In the published news and highlights from the 1930 biennial convention, there was no indication that this amounted to a significant change for the organization. Instead, the proceedings' highlights contained copious notes about the fundraising activities of the association and its chapters. Male nurses were included quietly and without fanfare. The understated admission of male nurses reveals an important reality for men. Admission did little to change the fact that they were still very restricted in the opportunities to practice in the field, and their future was still uncertain when it came to professional treatment.

Although national professional membership became available to male nurses in 1930, their modest numbers did little to help alleviate the continued inequity they faced within nursing organizations and the vocation. According to census accounts in 1930, 5,452 men reported "trained nurse" as their occupation.[26] Until their addition to the ANA, they lacked any national unifying male body to fight and organize on their behalf. Instead, it was up to active male nurses in state nursing associations and nursing schools to lead the fight.[27] According to one male nurse activist, the "effort and achievement on the part of men and of those responsible for their leadership" was the only way to assure the "changing attitude of women in the nursing profession towards male nurses."[28] Still, whatever hopes male nurses had about greater opportunities because of their acceptance into such a large national nursing organization proved elusive. Unless the entire nursing profession altered its attitude and perceptions, little would change for men in nursing.

Male nurses were by no means the silent minority. They actively discussed and pursued job opportunities and recognition from a variety of nursing associations, educational institutions, and the United States government. In the mid-1930s, the *American Journal of Nursing* published a series of articles that examined the vocational and educational opportunities for male nurses. Written by nurses and doctors alike, the articles concluded that improvements in nursing education and work toward professionalization increased the number of men in the profession. Dr. J. Frederick Painton, for example, noted that "with the gradual progress of nursing from very humble beginnings to its present place among professions . . . men, real men, are invading women's own profession and making good."[29] Yet the job opportunities or even advanced educational opportunities for male nurses remained few. Registered nurses Frederick Jones and Frances Witte complained of the scarcity of jobs for men nurses. This was the result of limited opportunities for advancement. "The time is at hand when the male student and graduate must have the same educational advantages as the young women, if we are to assure the community of safe and intelligent nursing," Witte writes.[30] Male nurse educational opportunities then were directly linked to vocational opportunities and recognition. Even in positions wherein male nurses were welcomed—in industrial nursing or mental hospitals—graduate trained male nurses faced competition from graduate female nurses with advanced training and untrained male nurses. Improving male nurse recognition and access to advanced or inclusive training remained the key to equality among the sexes in nursing.

LeRoy Craig, a graduate of the McLean Hospital School of Nursing for Men in Waverly, Massachusetts, became a leading advocate and activist for men in the nursing profession. In 1914 he accepted the position of directing the Pennsylvania Hospital School of Nursing for Men. Pennsylvania Hospital had a long tradition of training nurses; its school of nursing for women opened in 1875 and quickly became an innovator in the field. Its new school for men, with Craig at its helm, took a radical new approach to training male nurses. Unlike other schools of nursing that trained men, it consisted entirely of men. Its director, superintendents, instructors, and student body were all men. It was its "own organization, [had] a separate [governing] policy, its own ideals, and traditions." It was distinct from the School of Nursing for women.[31] This was unusual because male nurse training and education were traditionally conducted under female leadership. Even at schools that trained only men, women often served in leadership and oversight roles.

Men at the Pennsylvania Hospital School received training not only in psychiatric nursing but also as general nurses with genitourinary specialties. The idea was to improve the overall training of male nurses, thus producing more competent, well-rounded nurses who, as registered nurses, Frances Witte later suggested, would, "deepen [male nurses'] sense of social responsibility."[32] Furthermore, the education of male nurses by male nurses was groundbreaking. One male nurse commented that it was an "idea" from which "come ideals." It would produce a quality of men "who were capable and ready to serve where a woman, for various reasons, cannot." In short, several male nurse leaders believed that the right training and education of male nurses improved the condition and position of male nurses in civilian society and would extend to male nurses greater opportunities in industry and the military.[33] This training also demonstrated that men were capable enough to perform as professional nurses.

Following their acceptance in the ANA, Craig, along with male and female nurse activists, urged other nursing organizations to pursue similar recognition. They saw the American Red Cross as an obvious place to push for broader acceptance and employment of male nurses. The American Nurses' Association and American Red Cross had a long cooperative relationship; the ANA even worked with the Red Cross to create the Red Cross Nursing Service, the registry of nurses available for emergencies and service in the armed forces nurse corps. This established the ANA and Red Cross, along with the National League of Nursing Education (NLNE) and National Organization of Public Health Nursing (NOPHN), as the most prominent nursing groups directing nursing policies and the public's perception of nurse care in the United States.[34] In 1934 male nurse supporters asked the board of directors of the ANA to appeal to the National Committee on Red Cross Nursing Service to change its policy excluding men nurses from the service.[35] The Red Cross Nursing Service had not only served as the staffing organization for Army and Navy Nurse Corps since before World War I, but it had also provided a number of community health classes focused especially on the health and well-being of women and children.[36] The committee returned the following reply: "Inasmuch as the Red Cross Nursing Service is the reserve of the Army and Navy Nurse Corps which are composed of woman nurses and for which male nurses would not be accepted, no change be made in the present requirement . . . Furthermore . . . other types of Red Cross Nursing Services . . . being restrictive in nature, are not able to utilize other than woman nurses."[37] The Red Cross's response appeared to be practical for the kinds of services they provided. However, their decision overlooked how much their services might expand with the inclusion of men. The public health nursing aspect, for example, could expand to include male nurses for long-term, male-focused healthcare.

Given its primary focus on staffing the Army and Navy Nurse Corps, the Red Cross could do little to change its decision regarding male nurses. However, the organization's comments reflected not only the stereotype but also the public conviction that nursing, especially general nursing, was no place for men. More troubling and disappointing about the response of the Red Cross was the continuing insistence that male nurses, regardless of training or experience, should remain in very limited areas and jobs within the field of nursing. This included jobs in mental and psychiatric hospitals and jobs as private-duty nurses or in industrial nursing. Teaching courses in the care of the sick or working as public health nurses under the auspices of the Red Cross remained closed to men nurses. After men successfully gained membership in the American Nurses' Association, one can assume that the failure to change the policy of the Red Cross was a setback for those campaigning for full and fair recognition as nurses.

Nurses who aspired to service within the Army or Navy Nurse Corps first had to enroll in the Red Cross Nursing Service. The refusal of the Red Cross to change its policy with regard to male nurses in 1935 left little room for men to maneuver for a place within either nurse corps. Nevertheless, male nurses continued to appeal for change in the policies of the Red Cross concerning the employment of men. Nor did they stop applying pressure to the American Nurses' Association to take a more forceful role in supporting men in nursing. As U.S. entry into World War II became more likely in the closing years of the 1930s, male nurses, similar to African American female nurses, became another group that nursing leaders turned to in their attempt to coordinate nursing resources. This in turn provided men nurses the opportunity to draw attention to their cause. Near the end of 1939, the Red Cross reconsidered its policy concerning men and agreed to allow male nurses to register with the Red Cross Nursing Service. Registration with the service, however, was not meant to enroll men nurses for service in the Army or Navy Nurse Corps. It would organize "properly qualified male nurses, who if needed by the Army or Navy will serve . . . as technologists for service auxiliary to the Army and Navy Nurse Corps." These men, according to the announcement, would in the "event of national emergency . . . be eligible for enrollment in the Army as non-commissioned officers." While the requirements for male and female nurses wishing to apply to the nursing service were similar, the *American Journal of Nursing* reminded readers that federal law limited the job opportunities—at least in the military—for men nurses.[38] However, the Red Cross also continued to ignore male nurses for the other services it provided to local communities.

A 1940 recruitment appeal for nurses demonstrated that the Red Cross had not changed its opinion that nursing and women were synonymous. The informational insert in the *American Journal of Nursing* made no mention of male nurses; instead, it used feminine pronouns to describe nurses and to recruit women. This strengthened the argument of male nurses that as long as "nurse" remained defined as "she," men would occupy an inferior status to female nurses.[39] The continued emphasis on nursing as the natural function of women pointed to a larger societal understanding that caregiving was a biological function of women that translated to professional nursing as the apparent domain of women.[40] This recruitment plan, coupled with the Red Cross's limited acceptance of male nurses, suggests that allowing male nurses to register with the Red Cross Nursing Service was an organizational tactic used to help the Red Cross figure out how many male nurses were available for service in the event of an emergency. Although the Red Cross noted in April 1940 that changes to the nursing service had been underway for more than a year, and the threat of war had no basis in the decision, within months the major national nursing organizations in the United States organized the Nursing Council for National Defense with the purpose of planning the place of nurses in the nation's defense.[41]

Preparation for war allowed men in the American Nurses' Association to also take a stronger stance on pushing for male nurse recognition. This was in no small part due to the campaigning of male nurses and to the strong participation of men in their state nurses' associations. In the late 1930s, for example, district branches of the New York State Nurses' Association began forming Men Nurses' Committees to increase membership and the professional activities of male nurses throughout the state. They were able to sponsor men nurse sessions at state nursing conventions and eventually sessions and even a dinner at the American Nurses' Association's biennial convention. These statewide activities translated into increased publicity for male nurses at the national nursing level. As a result, the ANA created the Men Nurses' Section at their 1940 biennial convention in Philadelphia.[42] The section's job was to address the needs and issues that specifically affected male nurses. This included encouraging a better public understanding and acceptance of men in nursing and pushing for the use and recognition of male nurses within the Nurse Corps of the Armed Forces.[43] Beyond amending their membership requirements in 1930 and petitioning the Red Cross in 1935 on behalf of male nurses, this was the first major recognition by the ANA that the difficulties faced by male nurses needed special attention from the organization.[44]

One of the section's first duties with regard to expanding opportunities for male nurses was to publicize the American Red Cross's new program to enroll male nurses. In his 1940 article "Opportunities for Men Nurses," LeRoy Craig acknowledged that the Red Cross Nursing Service offered one possibility for men wishing to nurse with the federal government.[45] While not admission to the armed forces' nurse corps, Craig and other nurses noted that the status of male nurses in 1940 was much better than it had been in the previous two decades. In short, there was, at the very least, a recognition by the military and Red Cross that male nurses were vital to healthcare in the United States. However, did this signify a broadening attitude on the work and place of male graduate nurses, or was it a result of circumstance? Craig hoped that "in justice to men nurses they [male nurses] . . . be assured of duties, rank, and pay comparable to that granted other professional individuals." Would male nurses perceive serving as "medical technician or technologist" an acceptable alternative for service in the Army and Navy Nurse Corps?[46]

Male Nurses and the Nation's Defense

Several alumni and state nursing associations initially approved of the Red Cross Nursing Service Program. At the very minimum it was an opportunity for men nurses to gain some recognition in the military. Even this small concession was denied to a small group of nurses who sought recognition while serving in France during World War I.[47] Individually, however, most men dismissed the decision by the Red Cross to enroll male nurses for service as medical technicians; they viewed the program as an unsatisfactory resolution to the question of military service for men nurses. Sandy F. Mannino, for example, questioned the distinction in the acceptance of male nurses only as medical technicians when men and women received similar training, when men had membership in all the national nursing organizations, and when they were eligible for registration in every state.[48] Registered nurse Nathaniel Wooding echoed the same sentiment in a letter to the surgeon general's office: "Forty-seven schools of nursing [admit] men students" and "men candidates [met] the same qualifications as do women."[49] Over the course of six months following the initiation of the Nursing Service Program, male nurses struggled to convince the War Department, nursing leaders, and President Roosevelt that the use of male nurses as enlisted men and noncommissioned officers amounted not only to discrimination against men but also defeated the purpose of the nurse corps.[50] The basic law of the ANC, Edward F. Perreault wrote to the president, was an "antiquated law" that should be "repealed, and in its place get one which gives men and women nurses equal opportunity in the military service."[51] Whether in peace or wartime, these men argued, male nurses should be serving their country as nurses with the same privileges provided female nurses, not fighting to attain the right to do so.

In the fall of 1940, Congress passed and the president signed into law the first peacetime draft in United States history. The Selective Service Act mandated that every able-bodied man between the ages of twenty-one and thirty-five register for service in the U.S. military.[52] As part of their draft registration, men described their training and work capabilities in order to give the War Department an idea about how their skills would most benefit the military. The Red Cross informed male nurses that by registering with the Red Cross Nursing Service first, they would ensure that their extensive experience and training placed them into positions within the Medical Department. In a memo from the office of the surgeon general, the Army Medical Department listed the occupational specialties and accompanying serial numbers it recommended be assigned to the department when men were classified under the draft. This memo further noted that the Red Cross maintained a list of men identified under the occupation of medical technician (male nurse) and serial number 123. As a result, men who did not register with the Red Cross Nursing Service risked assignment outside the medical department in jobs that may have little to do with their nurse training. Furthermore, the group advised men that registering with the nursing service brought additional benefits. This included promotion to technical sergeant, if there were vacancies, and the eventual possibility of Officers' Candidate School after four months of training and service.[53]

This plan for the promotion of male nurses, however, proved problematic for several reasons. First, while many nursing leaders believed that the Red Cross and War Department's plan for male nurses was the first step to eventual acceptance of men into the Army Nurse Corps, not all men registered with the Red Cross. Registration with the Red Cross, although encouraged, was voluntary, and many men were suspicious that the program offered men little in the way of equality with female nurses. In fact, some male nurses refused to register as a means of protest. In a letter to Senator Henry C. Lodge, Mitchell Blake angrily noted, "I have been criticized . . . for not joining the Red Cross Service [but will not do so until] those of us who wished to devote our services can do so without reservation—and without doing the work of a hospital orderly."[54] Blake's terse remarks reveal the general sense of disgust that many male nurses felt at the blatant disregard for their training. Furthermore, in the summer before the bombing of Pearl Harbor, the Nursing Service counted only twenty-five men among their new enrollments.[55] Many male nurses believed that by not registering with the Red Cross Nursing Service, they had more control over where they would end up if drafted. Second, while male nurses wanted guarantees to advancement and possibly officer's status, the War Department stated that promotion would occur only if vacancies existed in particular ranks. This meant that registering with the Red Cross Nursing Service was no guarantee of better standing in the Army Medical Department or even assignment within it. Finally, because there was no guarantee of promotion for male nurses with nursing degrees or training, in some cases men with limited training as medics received promotion before men with civilian nursing degrees. If the War Department was so concerned with the best healthcare for their soldiers, why not allow men to join the ANC or, at the very least, as some suggested, form a sub-branch of the nurse corps focused on the specialties of male nurses? As a matter of fact, LeRoy Craig suggested the formation of a "reserve group of male nurses with psychiatric training with the rank of second lieutenant," the same rank initially given to female nurses. He believed that such a group would be able to address the psychological needs of soldiers and would provide some compensation to male nurses restricted from the nurse corps. However, he received little in the way of support from the surgeon general for his suggestion.[56]

The War Department and surgeon general's office responded to these suggestions by focusing on the impracticality of employing male nurses, an argument also used to limit African American female nurse participation. Replying to the American Nurses' Association's push to revoke the law that designated the ANC as a female institution and to include male nurses, Brigadier General Albert G. Love noted:

> I regret that this office cannot concur in your opinion. It would be impracticable to employ male nurses in time of peace since such employment could complicate unnecessarily the administrative problems. We feel that we have provided a satisfactory and dignified position for such male nurses as may be employed during the military emergency. In addition, we feel sure that the Secretary of War would not approve the legislation suggested by you.[57]

The administrative issues to which Love and others referred to centered on the impracticality of building separate housing and mess facilities and on the presumption that men nurses were soldiers first and nurses second.[58] Focusing on the "problems" involved in reversing the forty-year-old law mandating that only females work in the Army Nurse Corps, the surgeon general's office dismissed the subject of discrimination, which was in the forefront of the minds of many male nurses. Further, Love's assertion that the secretary of war would not approve of any changes to the current law and arrangement of the nurse corps suggests a genuine lack of support for any change. Love implied that to pursue such a course was unpatriotic and also in opposition to the war effort. Men and women each had a role, clearly delineated by sex; frontline activities were the responsibilities of men, while support and caregiving were the responsibilities of women.

This perspective on gender difference in the context of wartime recruitment raised uncomfortable questions about the responsibilities and obligations of male nurses in war mobilization before and after the bombing of Pearl Harbor in December 1941. Were they nurses or soldiers? Where did male nurses serve their country best, as civilians or in the military? According to Richard Musser, graduate male nurses best served their country doing their job for American soldiers. They, Musser argued, "expect to assume their part of the country's defense with the rest of the men . . . [but] their proper place in national defense is denied them."[59] This duty remained out of their reach because nursing—as the Red Cross recruitment campaign revealed—remained a female occupation. "Male" and "nurse" did not belong together. Overcoming this dichotomy was an ongoing struggle for male nurses, one that a particular nurse training school attempted to address two decades before the war by advertising their school as an institution that produced "men who think straight and see straight, who are capable and ready to serve where women, for various reasons, cannot."[60] The undertone in comments such as this stressed the difficulties male nurses faced in their chosen profession, especially during wartime. Already facing unfair treatment because of their sex, they had to persuade the American public of the importance, legitimacy and, to a large degree, the "manliness" of men nurses. While men nurses and their supporters could agree that assigning eligible men to military duty outside the nurse corps was a poor use of the workforce, some argued that the men nurses should be recruited instead to civilian hospitals to supplement the shortage of female nurses entering military service.

The Men Nurses' Section of the American Nurses' Association pushed this belief further by suggesting that the experience and training of male nurses should classify them as "necessary men" in war labor plans. Necessary men were those designated by the War Department as exempt from Selective Service because of the nature of their job. A man qualified for the classification if he met one of the following conditions: "he cannot be replaced satisfactorily because of a shortage of persons with his qualifications or skill in such an activity," or "his removal would cause a material loss of effectiveness in such activity." Furthermore, a necessary man was one in "any industry, business, employment, agricultural pursuit, governmental service, or . . . in training or preparation therefore, the maintenance of which is essential to the national health, safety, or interest in the sense that a serious interruption or delay in such activity is likely to impede the National Defense Program." According to nursing leaders, based on the War Department's own criteria, male nurses were "necessary men." The removal of male nurses from nursing schools by drafting them could have detrimental consequences for the future of nursing and impeded the ability of male nurses to do their jobs, thereby affecting national health.[61] If the military did not want them in the nurse corps, they were certainly essential in civilian hospitals. The surgeon general's office did not, however, agree with this assessment and responded that nothing in the Selective Service Act defined "male nurses as an occupational group."[62]

The National Nursing Council for War Service (NNCWS) bolstered the claim that men nurses could provide a valuable service to civilian life if the War Department had no intention of employing them as nurses.[63] Male nurses could be recruited, the council argued, to serve in civilian hospitals to replace the female nurses who joined the military or were recruited to care for American soldiers once they returned to the United States. The suggestion that men nurses support the war effort in this way was reminiscent of the strategy used to recruit women into the military and war industries.[64] While the public remained uncomfortable with and perhaps even suspicious of male nurses, the National Nursing Council for War Service argued that their labor was critical to the health of the civilian population and to the continuation of nursing programs.[65] Regardless of the NNCWS's comments, many men nurses understood that until the War Department changed its opinion on the use of them within the ANC, they could achieve no hope of parity in their civilian lives or the nursing profession. This understanding placed white male nurses in an unusual position; they found that their sex hindered their success in nursing even while they tried to serve their county. In this way, white male nurses, very much like African American female nurses—albeit for different reasons—saw military service as the first step in resolving claims of discrimination.

Very little changed for male nurses in the first two-and-a-half years of the war; with few exceptions, public discourse about nursing remained focused on the recruitment of women while the military judiciously avoided appeals from male nurses. Male nurse advocates, who included among their ranks the American Nurses' Association and the American Medical Association, were baffled about how to change the War Department's, surgeon general's, and Congress's opinion of trained male nurses.[66] Frustrated, male nurse R. A. Chiniok wrote: "I hope somebody can show the Washington legislators whereby the folly of the forty year law banning us out of the rights in Army Nursing."[67] The War Department, however, faithfully replied to all queries that during wartime male nurses "are not normally used by the Medical Department in times of peace," but they are used in accordance with provisions of the Selective Service Act: as medical technicians and orderlies.[68] Even without the provisions of the Selective Service Act to support their position, the War Department and surgeon general had a recent and ongoing tradition by which to set the example concerning the successful employment of male nurses in the U.S. military.

The U.S. Navy's special need for shipboard medical service led it down a path that produced male medical personnel with pharmaceutical, nursing, and general medical capabilities. In 1917 the U.S. Navy established the Pharmacist's Mate School. Here, men received instruction in a variety of subjects, including nursing and general healthcare, in preparation for duty with the hospital corps. As part of the hospital corps, pharmacist mates helped maintain the health of naval personnel and aided in the sick and disabled. In contrast to the women of the Navy Nurse Corps, however, these men also performed all manner of scientific work, became public health officers, served as independent medical officers on ships, drilled and instructed recruits, and assisted in clerical work. In other words, beyond their medical education, the pharmacist's mates received training in all aspects of military life. The pharmacist's mate was the epitome of the masculine nurse, one that removed almost all of the feminine traits of caregiving. By 1927 the Pharmacist's Mate School claimed for itself the title of "largest school for male nurses in the world." The fact that two states, California and Virginia, allowed graduates of the school to register as nurses supported this claim. The War Department and surgeon general then could and did use the U.S. Navy pharmacist's mate as an example on how to use men nurses in the current conflict in both the hospital corps and the army medical corps and avoid the charge of work discrimination. In doing so, however, they disregarded two points of contention among trained professional nurses: their education and their nursing experience before entering military service.[69] Moreover, the War Department's acceptance of female nurses as officers in the nurse corps and male nurses as privates in the Medical Department further provoked a sense of discrimination and lack of fair play among men nurses. It was made glaringly obvious to male nurses that neither their experience nor their education could ever overcome the fact that they were not women and therefore had no place in the ANC.

Col. Florence A. Blanchfield, chief of the Army Nurse Corps in 1943, argued that the corps would not be a satisfactory place for men within the military. "Our standing is not as good and in some respects not as secure," she wrote John Welch of the New York State Nurses' Association. Female nurse officers only carried a rank "relative" to the regular Army, without many of the same benefits as commissioned officers.[70] Historically, the matter of rank plagued the nurses' place in the military. When the ANC was founded in 1901 as part of the Army Reorganization Act, the act made no reference to either the rank or status of nurses. At the turn of the century, Congress and army leadership were reluctant to assign official rank or status to women in the military, even if they were nurses. Therefore, the only stipulations that defined the job and organization of the ANC were that the nurse corps would consist of a "superintendent, chief nurses, nurses, and reserve nurses." The surgeon general approved the appointment of the nurses to serve for three years. From the beginning, this vague definition presented problems for the ANC, especially the question of rank. Lack of clearly defined status and rank with the U.S. Army exposed nurses to abuse and unfair treatment not only from the Army Medical Department but also from the military establishment as a whole. As a result, by the end of World War I the army could no longer ignore the question of rank.[71]

Nurses and their supporters demanded equality in the form of official recognition in the U.S. Army. In June 1920 Congress reluctantly agreed, and President Wilson signed a bill that provided army nurses with "relative rank," or rank comparable to other officers. But even this came with limitations; the secretary of war defined exactly what relative rank meant for army nurses. Army nurses would be accorded the same respect and protection as other commissioned officers, including the right to wear the insignia of their grade and the privilege of salute, but would be denied the right to command, for example.[72] By 1943 the only change to this status was a 1942 bill that finally gave nurses pay commensurate with that of other commissioned officers. Even then, nurses were not entitled to be spoken to by rank but were supposed to be addressed as "nurse," according to Blanchfield. Therefore, incorporating male nurses into the ANC would have provided men with an empty title and only a temporary place in the military.[73] The underlying implication from this situation was that male nurses would want the same benefits granted to men in other positions in the military. The desired status would include the security of access to benefits to support their families, retirement, and career advancement. These discussions reveal how men's service alongside women in a female-gendered occupation could potentially create unacceptable inequalities between men and women in the nurse corps and among men in other military services. "No doubt men with relative rank would be more conscious of this difference in status than women are," Blanchfield surmised. In order to avoid this uncomfortable situation, the Medical Department assured male nurses that it kept them out of the nurse corps and assigned them to positions with the regular army in the "best interest of registered male nurses."[74]

A long tradition of gender segregation in nursing complicated the integration of men. Interestingly, the Medical Department and Colonel Blanchfield's assertion that male nurses needed protection from unequal treatment in the

ANC highlights the hypocrisy of the treatment of female nurse officers who received rank comparable only to commissioned male officers. In effect, the army denied women the full benefits and security of military service; accepting male nurses into the ANC would require that the army acknowledge this discrepancy and thereby be forced, perhaps, to consider equal treatment for women. By focusing on the reasons that male nurses should be denied entry into the ANC, army representatives shifted the spotlight away from gender inequality, but this did not diminish male nurses' hopes that the need for nurses would supersede gender discrimination.

The National Nursing Council for War Service (NNCWS) demonstrated the difficult nature of the male nurse campaign for ANC membership. As noted in chapter 2, African American female nurses secured an advantage when the NNCWS made their integration campaign a priority after mid-1943. Seeing African American women as a logical, but also severely underused, source of nursing power, the NNCWS took an active role in ending discriminatory quotas and treatment of black nurses. After researching the treatment of black nurses the year before, in early 1945 the NNCWS published its report, which revealed the damage done to the war effort and to the health and safety of American soldiers by neglecting to use African American female nurses more fully within the nurse corps.[75] The report claimed that a more inclusive use of eight thousand available African American female nurses would alleviate any shortage of nurses. Yet, not surprisingly, the report ignored the use of male nurses to meet nursing needs. This oversight reflected the differences in support and strategies that white male nurses and African American female nurses used in their integration campaigns. African American female nurses, with the help of the NNCWS, relied not only on the rhetoric of women's natural affinity to nursing to make their case, but they also looked to a well-organized advocacy group in the National Association of Colored Graduate Nurses that had long fostered connections to civil rights groups, politicians, and philanthropists. The report concluded that increasing the number of African American nurses would "demonstrate that as American men, regardless of race, creed, or color are fighting for democracy, American women are being given the opportunity, equally without discrimination, to care for them when ill or wounded."[76] Male nurses, in contrast, had only the Men Nurses' Sections in their State Nursing Associations, the newly formed Men Nurses' Section of the ANA, a few select politicians, individual nurses, and the lingering hope that legislation would change their predicament.

The Men Nurses' Section of the American Nurses' Association acted to publicize and campaign on behalf of male nurses. In December 1943, the section published an article in the *American Journal of Nursing*, which revealed that at least 320 graduate male nurses were serving with the armed forces in 1943 and another two thousand were available for service. While "a large proportion of the men nurses . . . [could have been] assigned to services where their nursing experience [could] be used," they were not, and therefore the "nursing and medical service has lost these men nurses who could have made a valuable contribution." Placing this article alongside the NNCWS's report, the failure to mention male nurses in the report is significant for two reasons. First, the number of male nurses in the armed forces was just ten less than the number of African American female nurses serving in the nurse corps, and yet the council seemingly ignored that the recruitment of men into the ANC could help reduce the nursing shortages that they argued harmed American soldiers. Second, the NNCWS's report failed to highlight that nearly 50 percent of the nursing shortage—based on the number of African American female and white male nurses available—would disappear with the use of both these groups. The goal of the Men's Section article was to "secure as much information as possible . . . [which] will be extremely useful when and if legislation is introduced"; however, the NNCWS's failure to use this information in its report just a year after the information on male nurses was published is telling. The NNCWS and its report portrayed nursing as a quintessentially female profession, even in the face of nursing shortages.[77]

Legislating Acceptance?

The integration of men into the ANC or, at the very least, rank and recognition of men as nurses was the central goal for male nurses throughout the war. Even before nursing shortages became a concern for both civilian and military officials, a growing movement of individuals called for legislation that would commission male nurses into the nurse corps and end the ANC's female-only directive. Nurses supported, and at least two national healthcare associations passed, early resolutions supporting a change in the status of male nurses. In two separate declarations, the American Nurses' Association and the American Hospital Association sought acknowledgment of male nurses from the U.S. Armed Forces. In 1942 the ANA adopted a resolution at the meeting of their house of delegates, whereby they requested that the surgeon general give men the "opportunity to serve as nurses as soon as possible after induction or enlistment." It is significant that the ANA did not ask for immediate male admission to the nurse corps, only that men serve as nurses in the armed forces. The ANA understood that the first step in pushing for parity between male and female nurses was not to demand the immediate acceptance of male nurses into the ANC. Removing the barriers to the ANC would come in gradual steps; recognition by the Medical Department needed to come first. A few months later, the American Hospital Association echoed this sentiment and adopted a more forceful resolution in light of increasing medical needs. They approved a recommendation to the War Department that male nurses receive the "same status in the Army as graduate female nurses."[78]

Beginning in early 1944, support for male nurses grew following the introduction of a series of legislative bills to Congress. That spring, Congresswoman Frances P. Bolton, long a proponent of nursing, introduced a bill to commission female nurse corps officers into the regular army. Nearly a year after members of the Women's Army Corps gained full army status as commissioned officers, members of the ANC remained under the vague designation of relative rank.[79] As part of her bill, Bolton suggested the removal of "female" from the current law governing the ANC as a way to ensure no further discrimination against female nurses and as a way to remove the barriers to the inclusion of male nurses. Had the bill passed as Bolton had first suggested, male nurses would have gained their first real victory in their struggle for equality. After all, it would be difficult—after the removal of the word "female" from the law—for either the War Department or the surgeon general to keep men out of the nurse corps without appearing prejudicial. The original bill was defeated, but a modified version drafted by the War Department did pass. The president signed H.R. 4445 into law on June 22, 1944, without removing the word "female" from the existing nurse corps law. Bolton relayed her disappointment to Technician Joseph Guerra: "I am well aware of the problems you are faced with and think the Army and Navy very unwise in their refusal to use your trained services to full capacity. . . . I am particularly troubled that we have not been able to make a dent in the situation." Having successfully remedied "the situation for the women," Bolton acknowledged six months later that since the president supported the idea of drafting nurses, "I am reorganizing my troops for a frontal attack" on the acceptance of male nurses.[80]

In May 1944, Congressman Thomas Lane of Massachusetts introduced H.R. 4760, a bill to grant commissions to male nurses, to the Committee on Military Affairs for discussion. A month later, at the American Nurses' Association's annual conference in Buffalo, New York, the organization passed a resolution supporting commissions for male nurses in the ANC. Given the legislative discussions, the backing of the ANA, and most especially the growing concern about the nursing shortage, male nurses' hope for a significant change in their situation did not appear at all unrealistic.[81]

Two situations shifted the male nurse campaign in the public debate. First, in June 1944 female nurse officers gained commissioned status in the regular army for the duration of the war and for six months after.[82] No longer were they auxiliary officers with the military; they were military women. This meant that for at least while the war continued, the army could no longer insist that the nurse corps did not provide security or mobility for male nurses. At the very least, male nurses argued, allow them to serve as nursing specialists in psychiatric or urological areas. It was precisely from this argument, however, that Surgeon General Kirk articulated his true feeling on male nurses. "It is believed . . . that the female nurse is, in general, more adaptable, competent, and reliable than the male nurse . . . male nurses do not get the broad training given female nurses, and . . . they are equally limited in the scope of their professional experience in civilian hospitals."[83] At the heart of this comment was the general belief in the inferiority of male nurses, not because they lacked training in general nursing—by 1940 most training schools for men trained them in general nursing—but because they lacked comprehensive training that included obstetrics and gynecology. Even the American Nurses' Association, however, acknowledged the substitution of genitourinary training for membership within the professional organization. The surgeon general's oversight on the training of male nurses aside, Kirk's shortsightedness speaks more about the inability to see a nurse as anyone but a woman and a failure to acknowledge that nursing soldiers did not necessitate the skills that differentiated female and male nurses in the civilian profession. Kirk ended his comments by stating, "There are relatively few places in the Army where the particular abilities of the male nurse are needed, and for these positions the Army has provided appropriate noncommissioned grades."[84] Essentially, the War Department and surgeon general affirmed that, regardless of training, education, or experience, male nurses' acceptance in the ANC would never happen.

Second, and even more pressing for the male nurse campaign, was the increasing shortage of nurses. While debates raged about the true nature of the nursing workforce, a large segment of the American population believed that the nursing shortage was growing progressively worse as the war continued.[85] Army recruitment campaigns, aiming to enlist one thousand new nurses each month in the summer of 1944, supported this contention. The army and War Department even announced the decision to increase the number of black nurses serving with the ANC in July 1944 in an attempt to alleviate shortages. While African American leaders heralded this moment as a significant strike to end discrimination against black female nurses, this move did little to ease the shortages or increase the number of black female nurses accepted into the Army Nurse Corps.[86] This became abundantly clear to Surgeon General Norman T. Kirk when in December 1944 he sent a number of "general hospitals overseas without nurses." It was this predicament, coupled with worries about the ability to care for both the civilian population and fighting men, that led the surgeon general to announce that drafting female nurses might be necessary even while he rejected proposals to accept men into the ranks of the ANC. Roosevelt's announcement before Congress supporting a female nurse draft in January 1945 was not well received by the general public. Many feared that drafting not only women but women in a single occupation set a dangerous precedent and one that was unnecessary if the military, particularly the army, took advantage of a valuable resource in African American female and white male nurses.[87]

By the beginning of 1945 the decision to introduce a bill designed to draft nurses weakened arguments against having males in the ANC. Writing to Congresswoman Bolton, male nurse Robert Cincotta stated: "While the Army is crying for more nurses, it is overlooking thousands of male RNs at its own doorstep. Can something be done about that?"[88] The surgeon general's office, however, remained firm in its belief that women were best suited to serve in the nurse corps. As to the use of male nurses, Surgeon General Norman Kirk again demonstrated that gender was the key factor in the War Department's support of drafting female nurses instead of men. Kirk stated that female nurses were "appointed for a single, specific duty for which they are particularly qualified by reason of their sex. . . . Army nurses of either sex must accord patients all the usual care required by duties of their profession, including a variety of intimate offices and quasi-menial services. Women of officer rank can render those duties without incongruity, while men of such rank could not."[89] Women officers were better qualified on the grounds of perceived gender identities and their assumed ability to provide the menial services—such as general housekeeping, emptying bedpans, and so forth—that doctors and hospitals had expected from them for decades. Male officer nurses would be able to provide basic care for soldiers but would still be restricted from providing care to women and/or children. Furthermore, according to Rear Admiral W. J. C. Agnew, enlisted men in the hospital corps—the navy equivalent of the army medical corps—were called on to carry out many more duties beyond those involving nursing, whereas female nurses were not. Obtaining officer's rank in the hospital corps meant performing duties "almost entirely . . . of an administrative nature"; therefore, seldom (if any) nursing duties.[90] In light of such knowledge, the War Department remained committed to an all-female nursing corps. Moreover, it was within this atmosphere that Kirk admitted the necessity of drafting female nurses to meet nursing shortfalls in late 1944, and President Roosevelt's decision to support this idea in January 1945.

Male nurses found it difficult to win recognition that they, too, were a viable option in avoiding a female draft. While nursing leaders such as Katherine Densford and Congresswoman Bolton supported the idea of commissioning and using male nurses in the military, most male nurses felt generally ignored. As one male nurse pointed out, "The male nurse is left out in the cold. . . . Can one honestly say that there is a nursing shortage in an Army which drafts male R.N.'s to work in kitchens, or fix a plane, or march in the infantry?"[91] These feelings did not stop male nurses from inundating, with telegrams and letters, the offices of Congresswomen Bolton, Edith Nourse Rogers, and others in the wake of Roosevelt's announcement. One male nurse from Texas declared: "Ten thousand Nurses Available. Nurses Draft Unnecessary."[92] While a letter from a female superintendent of nursing read: "In view of the serious shortage of nurses, cannot some way be found to use the *male nurses* who are now in the service . . . there must be 1000–2000 of them."[93] Certainly, by January 1945, the public was well versed in the possibility of using male nurses to alleviate the shortage. Nevertheless, neither Congress nor the military did much to facilitate the acceptance of male nurses. Frances Bolton recognized that "the Army Nurse Corps was created as a 'female' Corps, and there is a very strong feeling that it would be exceedingly unfortunate to change that fundamental ruling."[94]

Testimony before the Military Affairs Committee reveals that the possibility of using male nurses was not far from the minds of those in attendance. Congresswoman Bolton even attempted to introduce another bill granting male nurses commission. Like her previous efforts and those of Congressman Thomas Lane, the new bill did not reach the debate stage. Instead of supporting this legislation, the War Department decided to end all restrictions keeping African American female nurses from joining the ANC in early 1945. The ANC would now accept, without regard to race, all qualified female nurses.[95] This was a major victory for African American female nurses, but it proved just the opposite for male nurses. While many did not like the idea of drafting women into the military, citizens seemed even less comfortable with accepting male nurses as caregivers to soldiers and their families. In February, the National Opinion Research Center surveyed a "cross-section" of white adults about receiving care from a black nurse. It revealed that 57 percent of participants believed that receiving care from an African American nurse would be acceptable.[96] The poll's emphasis on the public's acceptance of female nurses, regardless of their race, made no mention of male nurses; in doing so, it highlighted an important point about the nursing shortage and nurse draft: nursing was a female occupation and obligation.

Nurse draft legislation did not vanish with the surgeon general's declaration accepting all female nurses into the ANC. The congressional debates over the issue ensued for months. Representative Andrew J. May even managed to bring House Resolution 2277, as a revision of the original Nurse Draft Bill, H.R. 1284, before the House on March 5, 1945.[97] The revised bill defined which nurses were subject to the draft. The draft would include only unmarried women between the ages of twenty and forty-five who were registered nurses and graduates of nursing schools eligible for certification. It exempted any nurse who was deemed essential in her current job.[98] Proponents, including some of the staunchest supporters of African American female and white male nurses, believed that the draft of female nurses was the first step to a more complete Selective Service Act that would ensure adequate military support for years to come and include all citizens. Opponents of the proposed legislation believed it to be too one-sided in its approach because it singled out one specific occupational cross-section—the majority of which was populated by women—for selective service.[99] The House of Representatives passed an amended version of H.R. 2277 that included the addition of a discrimination clause that added "sex" among the qualifications that could not obstruct a nurse from the draft, before sending it to the Senate for final approval. The Senate asked for clarification on a number of provisions, including the discrimination clause as it pertained to male nurses. Then, after months of debates, the surgeon general quietly announced to nurse leaders on May 24, 1945, that "no further action was to be undertaken" regarding draft legislation. The Senate had "passed over" the bill. They abandoned the bill because nearly twenty-five thousand women volunteered in answer to President Roosevelt's appeal for nurses, and the war was nearing its end. Thus, the War Department avoided the question of the constitutionality of a female draft and closed the debate about the inclusion of male nurses in the ANC.[100]

Shifting attitudes regarding race and gender relations marked World War II even while many Americans continued to embrace traditional values. While the exigencies of war refashioned women's duties in the workforce, albeit temporarily in some cases, they did not alter all responsibilities and obligations gendered as male or female. The result was that although the possibility of drafting female nurses helped to end race restrictions in the ANC, but not race discrimination, it also perpetuated discrimination against male nurses in both the military and civilian society. For male nurses, gender became the important factor in determining who was best suited to provide care to America's fighting men. Frances Bolton's response to a male nurse underscored the general belief that the admission of male nurses to the ANC would overturn the gender norms of the profession: "The Army Nurse Corps was created as a 'female' Corps, and there is very strong feelings that it would be exceedingly unfortunate to change that fundamental ruling, not because men can't nurse well and are not really desperately needed in some of the specialties, but rather because men as a whole do better with women nurses than men."[101] Repeatedly, when faced with questions about male nurses, the War Department reiterated traditional beliefs about gender roles—even when faced with desperate nursing shortages.

Nevertheless, the debates about men nurses and the gender restrictions within the Army Nurse Corps did not fade away. Nursing shortages persisted and continued to be a problem for the nurse corps and for civilian society. They remained tied to a larger discussion about discrimination and equality in the postwar period. Cold War fears and a growing civil rights campaign forced the armed forces to refashion its fighting force; it addressed not only race, but also gender roles in its attempt to meet the challenges it faced in its fight to defend democracy. While the question about whether soldiers worried about the race or sex of the nurse providing care was provocative, it did not change the fact that, in the end, the sex of the nurse did matter to some people. Both the military and civilian society at large ultimately supported the idea that nursing was the responsibility of women, not men. Sex, rather than race, proved to be the overriding determinant of who could nurse during World War II.

4

An American Challenge

Defense, Democracy, and Civil Rights after World War II

In a period of defense, it is futile to protect democracy
from without while destroying it from within.[1]

—Margaret Culkin Banning, *American Journal
of Nursing*, December 1951

In the ten years following World War II, professional nursing viewed its responsibilities to the health and welfare of the nation as being bound to the global defense of democracy. Nursing became part of the "frontline" in maintaining America's strength against the disease of communism. To maintain this "frontline" successfully, nursing leaders looked inward and used perceived Cold War threats to mobilize and improve the profession for national security. Civilian nursing groups, including the American Nurses' Association (ANA) and the National Organization of Public Health Nursing (NOPHN), set about resolving what they framed as two of the greatest threats to democracy in the United States: unequal access to healthcare and discrimination in the workplace. Nursing groups also associated the nation's future health and well-being with their ability to foster cooperation among all nurses without regard to race, sex, creed, or ethnicity. The only way to safeguard the nation's future health was to guarantee the integration and cooperation of all nurses in the profession. The influence of World War II on traditional gender roles and race relations did affect nursing, albeit in contradictory ways. In the postwar period, the ongoing effects of World War II figured prominently in the nursing profession, especially in the ANC as they grappled with their new role in a military engaged in new and unfamiliar wars.

The continuing efforts to integrate the ANC reflected the events, activities, and fears that materialized in civil society following World War II. The story of the ANC during this period is a complex web of overlapping gendered successes and failures, expanded economic opportunities, and racial challenges. Conservative anticommunist fervor promoted setbacks to New Deal era and World War II gains and revealed the complicated nature of equality in American society.[2] Increasing attention on civil rights in the context of the early Cold War and later Korean War placed new burdens on the ANC. The integration of African American female nurses and the transformation of the nurse corps into a permanent member of the Army Medical Department in 1947 did not end discrimination and exclusion in the ANC. Racial segregation in civilian society still affected day-to-day interactions in the United States military and, by extension, in the nurse corps. Traditional gender arrangements in the nursing profession also remained a difficult reality for male nurses to overcome. Yet the changing nature of war during the Korean hostilities led some to question the wisdom of holding tight to conventional values that saw gender as "an appropriate rationale for distributing work."[3] While most civilians and the military continued to cast nursing as female work, men nurses employed conventional rhetoric on gender roles to their advantage once the United States entered the conflict in Korea. This suggested, as was the case for African American female nurses earlier, that the quest for equal rights was a complicated negotiation between the use of traditional attitudes on gender expectations and the demand for a change to conventional beliefs on race and gender roles.

With the passage of the Army-Navy Nurse Act of 1947, female nurses achieved what had eluded women throughout the existence of the nurse corps: recognition as full military personnel with the benefits and professional future that came with it.[4] The enactment of the new law, however, was not without debate. Conversations on gender characteristics and racial discrimination weaved through public and congressional debates on the bill. Certainly, for female nurses, permanent inclusion in the military confirmed caregiving as a universally understood duty of women performed inside and outside the home.[5] Military service allowed women to provide an even greater service to the country, according to a recruitment article; the army nurse provided care for "the pick of the nation's manhood." As such, "no more rewarding opportunity to serve mankind . . . could be offered to American women," wrote one nurse corps colonel.[6] Yet what was the fervent acceptance of female nurses was also part of the ongoing rejection of male nurses and men's challenge to the belief that they had a role in caregiving.

The emphasis on American women caring for American men ignored the service of male nurses. As with Congresswoman Frances P. Bolton's 1944 commission bill, attempts to strike the word "female" from the existing law in 1947 met little favorable response in the postwar period.[7] Almost all could agree that nursing needed to be a permanent part of the Medical Department, but few supported the idea that both women and men should serve within its ranks. The refusal of Congress or the military to support the removal of "female" from the law in 1947 pointed to a continued refusal to recognize "nurse" as any gender but female. It meant that women could continue to foster their autonomy and authority in the nursing profession, something that they could rarely obtain in other occupations inside and outside the military. Furthermore, the integration of female nurses into the regular army and the decision to continue the Women's Army Corps indicated a change in the gendered culture of the U.S. military. The federal government and military recognized that the future sustainability of the armed forces required that women be permanent members of the military.[8] This was something that no citizen dared imagine before 1945. There would no longer be a time when women did not serve their country, albeit in noncombat jobs.

The Army-Navy Nurse Act of 1947 also reinforced the idea that discrimination and civil rights would remain an important part of political and social discussions about the military and civilian society in the postwar period. During the congressional debates of the act, Representative Adam Clayton Powell introduced the Powell Amendment, an antidiscrimination amendment to the bill intended to safeguard against any discrimination in the employment of African American female nurses. This would make permanent a similar amendment that had passed in 1945 as part of the temporary legislation on nurses. Ultimately, the Powell Amendment was defeated; Representatives Frances Bolton and Margaret Chase Smith had successfully argued that the amendment was unnecessary, as the bill did not "prohibit the employment of Negro nurses, but leaves recruitment entirely to the discretion of the army and navy leaders." While this sentiment echoed both the Jim Crow and "separate but equal" mentality concerning the treatment of African Americans in the United States, it failed to recognize the importance of discrimination in nursing to a wider civil rights struggle. In reflecting on the amendment's defeat at least one newspaper reported, for example, that the House Republican majority worried, in hindsight, that they would lose African American voting support in the upcoming election as a result.[9]

Black Activism in Early Cold War Defense

Civil rights activists and African American organizations emerged from World War II reenergized in their push for equality. Black Americans had successfully "exploited World War II to improve the material conditions and

civil rights of the black community."[10] They accomplished this by manipu-
lating the mantra of "freedom, democracy, and equality," which the Allies
used to unite their forces during World War II.[11] On the surface, this strategy
appeared to work, as black Americans obtained jobs in wartime industries,
gained recognition in the military, and even managed to win a significant
political victory with the abolition of white primaries.[12] Black participation
in the military provided hope for the future of black men and women.[13] African American female nurses could even boast that the ANC desegregated
before the end of the war in 1945 and integrated into the military a year before
President Truman signed his executive order in 1948, when Congress passed
the Army-Navy Nurse Act in 1947. These wartime victories, however, did not
translate easily into opportunities in postwar American society.

Indeed, during World War II racial violence accompanied civil rights successes in equal measure. Tensions over the availability of jobs and housing
generally, together with the migration of African Americans to defense-
industry cities where the population of minorities grew quickly, resulted
in a number of violent race riots that plagued the country throughout the
war. The bloodiest of these took place in Detroit in 1943.[14] While the nation
preached equality for all citizens, these riots pointed out how tenuous African
American gains and peaceful race relations were in the United States. At the
end of the war, returning black soldiers faced not the welcome of a grateful
nation. Instead, they met a nation divided over the role of African Americans
in postwar American society, and racial violence increased with particularly
violent acts directed at returning veterans.[15] In this context, growing Cold
War tensions and anticommunism undermined and yet strengthened the civil
rights movement by silencing some of the movement's most radical activists
while supporting a more moderate message of civil rights to the public.[16]

Postwar violence troubled civil rights organizations and activists because
they believed it undermined everything the country had fought to protect
during the war. In a series of public protests against racial violence during
the summer of 1946, picketers carried signs that read "Speak! Speak! Mr.
President" and "Where is Democracy?" They looked to the president—and
through him toward federal action—to address the violence and racial injustice.[17] Taking their cue from the March on Washington movement, the
protesters helped form the National Emergency Committee against Mob
Violence. The organization sought federal action to end the increasing violence against racial minorities, especially returning veterans. They met with
President Truman in late 1946 to demand he take concrete action against the
violence. Faced with the evidence of racial violence, a stronger civil rights
movement, and the strengthening Cold War, Truman had little choice. He

formed the President's Committee on Civil Rights (PCCR) in December 1946 and ordered the group to study the state of civil rights in the nation and to recommend steps for improving the civil rights of every citizen.[18]

Published in late 1947, the committee's report became politically important for President Truman and civil rights activists. The recommendations of the committee help set, according to one scholar, the "federal government's agenda on civil rights."[19] The mere existence of the PCCR helped to encourage civil rights activists to continue pushing the federal government to do more to ensure that the democratic tenets of the nation benefited all citizens. Civil rights organizations, such as the NAACP, the National Urban League, the National Association of Colored Graduate Nurses (NACGN), and the National Council of Negro Women, issued calls to Congress to enact legislation to support the committee's recommendations.[20] The report recommended that a number of measures be put in force to protect and expand civil rights in the United States a year before the next presidential election. Among them was the formation of a permanent Fair Employment Practices Committee and the immediate end to all discrimination and segregation in the armed forces based on race, color, creed, and national origin.[21] The possibility of reinstating the draft and the African American community's vehement opposition to another Jim Crow army forced Truman to take these two recommendations seriously. He understood that "waging the Cold War would require military strength" and national unity.[22] In early 1948, Truman took the first steps toward changing military policy by announcing his intentions to issue a policy of nondiscrimination toward any person serving in the United States Armed Forces.

Although Truman's plans met with some resistance from members of Congress and constituents, as well from as the military, he gained valuable support for his reelection from the black community. In issuing his Executive Order 9981, Truman wrote that it was "essential that there be maintained in the armed services of the United States the highest standards of democracy with equality of treatment and opportunity for all those who serve in our country's defense." Therefore, "race, color, religion, or national origin" would no longer determine a person's fitness in serving his country.[23] While Truman's executive order did not explicitly mention the words "desegregation" or "integration," many Americans read this intent in the order. For African Americans especially, this change in military policy was long overdue, one that many viewed as a necessary step to full equality, and civil rights activists used the language of desegregation or integration to promote what they hoped was the long-term result of the order.[24] The *Chicago Defender* heralded the order as a "dramatic and historic move, unprecedented since the time of

Lincoln."[25] It was also, however, a victory that would come at some cost for the larger civil rights movement.

Truman's order of nondiscrimination in the armed forces was a victory for African Americans. A. Philip Randolph had urged African Americans to boycott the reinstatement of the draft to protest ongoing racial discrimination in the military. The passage of Executive Order 9981 reiterated to Randolph that, as his March on Washington Movement had done during World War II, a unified black protest movement did produce change. Yet mounting Cold War tensions between 1946 and 1948, including the release of the Truman Doctrine and the Berlin blockade, changed the way the military could be used for protest.[26] Cold War tensions tolerated little dissent against the unity of the nation, and the Department of Justice even hinted that any further disruption in the draft could bring an investigation of individuals and groups.[27] The military would continue to be a platform to argue for equality, but civil rights activists could no longer point to a divided army as the most overt representation of racial injustice in the United States.

The passage of Executive Order 9981 in the summer of 1948 affected the ANC in a contradictory fashion. For African American female nurses, the act that would support the desegregation of the U.S. military merely reiterated a policy instituted late in World War II. Technically, by early 1945 the ANC had integrated because the Army had ended their quota policy and banned discrimination against African American female nurses. Truman's order meant an eventual end to segregated units and hospital staff—but not immediately, and certainly not an end to discrimination against racial minorities.[28] For African Americans the first test of this order came during the Korean War. Truman's executive order was even more curious in light of the ongoing male nurse campaign. Male nursing activists did not cite E.O. 9981 as a reason to end restrictions against male nurses in the Armed Forces Nurse Corps; however, there was a marked increase in their campaign after 1948. Several newspaper articles and letters suggest an escalation in the push for equal opportunity for male nurses in the nurse corps.[29] Truman's focus on the "equality of treatment and opportunity for all those who serve the nation" helped strengthen the case for male nurse inclusion, but so did a renewed commitment to equality in the civilian nursing profession.

The Anti-Discrimination Campaign of the ANA

In 1948 the American Nurses' Association founded the Intergroup Relations Committee. The committee's primary agenda focused on equal rights, particularly in the postwar period, and on the importance of men and minority female nurses to the future of the profession. Broadly defining its concern within the health of the nation, the American Nurses' Association linked continuing discrimination in the United States to a failure of its citizens to learn from and understand one another, and to guarantee economic security and labor protection to all nurses. This program confronted the foundation of the civil rights agenda that "understood economic security as essential to autonomy and justice."[30] Health, the group believed, was "more than the absence of disease or handicap, and true integration of minority groups in our culture must amount to more than the absence of segregation."[31] The committee, therefore, saw health and healthcare as a critical place to break down social and economic barriers to minority nurses, including male nurses, and to ensure the defense of the nation.[32] The nursing profession was not alone in linking the nation's defense to a more unified citizenry; the profession had taken its lead from postwar rhetoric on domestic security.

Although federal laws such as the Hill-Burton Act made nursing important to the healthcare system in the postwar period, nursing shortages made diversity in the profession even more important.[33] By 1950 the vision of the nursing profession from within its own ranks was vastly different than it had been ten years earlier. Take, for example, the illustration of a group of nurses singing carols printed in the *National News Bulletin* of the NACGN.[34] It was published in December 1950 as the NACGN was preparing to dissolve its organization and merge completely with the ANA. From the viewpoint of African American nurses, the illustration reveals a much more inclusive image of the nursing profession. Represented are white and African American female nurses, and a male nurse. The artist also included what appear to be Asian and Hispanic nurses. While this was an idealized or optimistic vision of the profession, the illustration does point to the fact that minority female nurses and male nurses were becoming more familiar to many in the public. Nursing census records indicate that more than three thousand African American female nurses and nine hundred male nurses enrolled in nursing schools in 1950.[35] The experiences of World War II, the Cold War, and continuing nursing shortages made the growing diversity of the nursing profession more noticeable and acceptable in civilian society. Nevertheless, male nurses in particular suffered an ongoing invisibility among hospital staffs, as their numbers remained low in most places that Americans received medical care. The struggle to overcome discrimination in its many forms remained a constant, however, as was revealed by the fact that an Intergroup Relations Committee was even necessary. Changing social attitudes did not

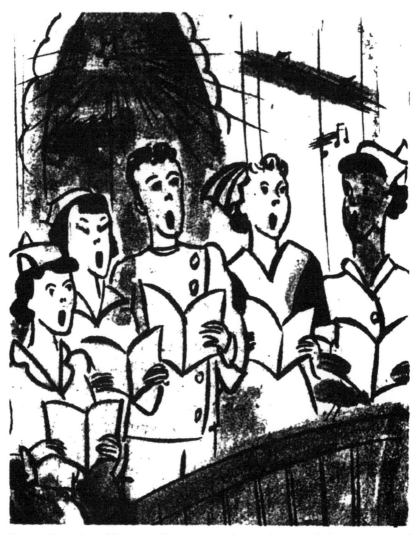

Figure 3. The author of this nurse illustration is unknown; however, the image was printed in the last issue of the *National News Bulletin* of the NACGN, just before the group dissolved and merged with the ANA. *National News Bulletin* 4, no. 2 (December 1950).

occur overnight but were the result of persistent struggles and failures. This was why the nursing profession's concentration on integration, as well as commentary like the one presented in the *National News Bulletin*, provided civil rights activists some tangible proof that their work was making a difference and could continue to do so.

The dissolution of the NACGN and the incorporation of African American women into the ANA was further evidence of the profession's growing connection to the civil rights movement and its goals.[36] After several years of discussion between the ANA and the NACGN, the ANA voted in 1948 for the full membership of black nurses. Backing their decision and commitment, they "appointed a black nurse as assistant executive secretary in the national headquarters and witnessed the election of Estelle Massey Osborne to the board of directors."[37] In January 1951, the NACGN voted, in turn, to dissolve their organization. In reflecting on the event, civil rights activist Judge William H. Hastie described it as the "dynamics of social evolution at its best."[38] Even famed poet Langston Hughes wrote a poem commemorating the successful work of black nurses:

> In the Army, the Navy, colored nurses attend.
> Her long gallant struggle portends a good end.
> "Negro nurse" is a phrase men no longer need say.
> "American nurse" means all nurses today.[39]

Members of the largest minority group fighting for equal rights in the country had gained an established place among one of the country's oldest nursing advocacy organizations. Without membership restrictions keeping some African American nurses from the ranks of the ANA, black nurses joined men nurses as full members of the ANA.[40] The strides that both groups made in the previous ten years were apparent in the number of schools available for their training and the expanding numbers of male and African American female nurses practicing in the profession.[41] The true test of these changes, however, came not in civilian hospitals but in the military of the United States as individuals, nurses, and soldiers alike attempted to serve and defend their nation.

The Pursuit of Equal Opportunity

The campaign to integrate men into the ANC gained strength from Cold War activities in the late 1940s and the reinstatement of the draft in March 1948. War between the United States and the Soviet Union became a near possibility at the end of the 1940s. These developments increased concerns about the availability of nurses but also fueled new rumors about a nurse draft.[42] In late 1949, the ANA notified the ANC of its intention to introduce and support legislation to permit the commissioning of male nurses.[43] Members of the Men Nurses' Section argued that the inclusion of men in the nurse corps was necessary to ensure an adequate reserve of care providers. The likelihood of a new war reinforced this argument. Furthermore, male nurse supporters added that the addition of men allowed the nurse corps flexibility in how they provided care and protected against placing women on front lines of battle. Nurse advocates hoped that, unlike previous attempts to integrate male nurses, the permanency of the nurse corps and the president's support of nondiscrimination in the armed forces would finally translate to success for their cause.

Female nurses tempered this hope. Col. Mary G. Phillips, chief of the ANC, responded to the ANA's announcement by soliciting opinions from her chief nurse officers regarding the possibility of including men into the ANC.[44] By early 1950 army nurse officers outlined a long list of the possible effects that inclusion of male nurses might have on their lives and work experiences.[45] There was plenty at stake for female nurses. Besides the Women's Army Corps, the nurse corps was the only area in the military dominated by women and was the place that women had carved out to participate in the nation's defense. As one nurse suggested, the ANA's move was "not much of a surprise, . . . [but] I am sure it is something we have all hoped would never really come up."[46] Her response reveals the trepidation that women felt about the inclusion of men in an occupation they had struggled to claim and professionalize as their own. Under other circumstances, the exclusion of men might be viewed as discrimination; however, the lack of opportunity for male nurses in the mid-twentieth century was part of what Alice Kessler-Harris termed the "gendered imagination." In this case, resistance to male nurses was perceived as "natural" because nursing was understood to be a female occupation. Sex discrimination was unacknowledged until the passage of the 1964 Civil Rights Act.[47] Nevertheless, discrimination was the term employed by male nurses to describe their own experiences within the profession without any acknowledgement to the historic discrimination faced by women in the work environment. By keeping male nurses out of the ANC, female nurses protected their jobs and economic security, but they also maintained social policies that constructed clearly defined identities between the sexes.

Female nurses expected only a few advantages from allowing men nurses in the ANC.[48] First, the majority of respondents agreed that men could fill existing vacancies in the corps. This would make the ANC more efficient; it would mean that during emergencies the military could use male nurses, especially in conflict zones in which, many believed, it was impossible for women to live and work. Second, female officers acknowledged that assigning male nurses to patients and offering specialized care that mirrored what they did in civilian hospitals would be advantageous to patients; this was something most doctors and nurses agreed on before 1950.[49] Some female nurses continued to believe that in at least two specialties—psychiatric nursing and genitourology—gender conventions suggested the preference for male nurses when possible. Finally, a small number of nurses acknowledged that there was no real reason male nurses should be restricted from joining the ANC. Certainly, their sex should not hamper their involvement in the care of male soldiers. Lt. Col. Ruby Bryant pointed out that the "majority of patients in Army hospitals are male patients"; therefore, "the sex of a nurse should be of no consequence so long as efficient nursing care is rendered."[50] While these opinions were definitely in the minority, the fact that even one nurse voiced them is interesting, given the prevailing ideals about gender characteristics and the nursing profession, particularly in the military. That a chief nurse willingly acknowledged that the sex of a nurse should not determine competency does suggest a nascent understanding that gender bias affected male nurses as well as female nurses.

Regardless of men's skills, however, female nurse objections, in contrast, clearly defended women's gains in a male-dominated milieu. Their objections also illuminate the conservative gender ideology underscoring much of the argument against the acceptance of male nurses. Female nurses were concerned not only about the loss of position and authority but also about the very tangible differences in the treatment of women and men serving in the armed forces. Organizationally, many female officers and the surgeon general rationalized that the addition of male nurses "would not be economical to the Army" or the government.[51] This was an argument posited by the U.S. military since the early years of World War II. Many of the nurse officers argued that it would mean changing legislation, adding housing for men, and paying dependency wages if the men were married or had children. All of this would be of tremendous expense to the government and the army. Further, many argued, the small number of men eligible for military service would ultimately become a burden to the nurse corps instead of a benefit.[52]

Most nurses also pointed out that men would be limited to duty in certain wards, while female nurses cared for all patients regardless of sex or circumstances.[53] So while male nurses perceived their possible inclusion in the ANC as a step forward in breaking down gender barriers across the profession, female nurse officers did not see men's inclusion as a move toward gender equity. This was true in large part because female nurses saw gender equity differently from how male nurses viewed the problem. In rejecting the addition of male nurses to the ANC, female nurse officers emphasized the organizational and legislative challenges of male nurse integration and reiterated their concern with the lost opportunities for female nurses.

Possible distinctions between duty assignments, responsibilities, and benefits alarmed female nurses. They framed these concerns as a morale factor in their list of the disadvantages to male nurse inclusion. Many of the officers believed that female nurses would become dissatisfied with serving in the ANC if men appeared to gain an advantage over them. This was a real possibility if, according to one nurse, one considers that the least attractive assignments—caring for women and obstetrics—would be the sole responsibility of women. Assignment to these areas meant monotony, little flexibility, and few opportunities to provide service across the ANC. Major Francis C. Gunn put it succinctly when she wrote, "Utilization of male nurses I feel is going to prove to be a source of annoyance to female nurses" and "will ultimately lead to dissatisfaction among the female nurses." Female nurses had worked hard for many of the benefits they received as members of the regular army, but inequities remained between men and women in all branches and departments of the military.[54]

As a single-sexed department, the ANC remained somewhat removed from the inequities between men and women service members. The addition of male nurses, however, had the potential of introducing two sets of laws and policies for the same organization. In the early postwar period, female nurses could not have dependent children under age eighteen, nor could they be married prior to joining the ANC. Those already serving in the ANC had to gain army approval to marry.[55] Women could not receive dependent pay unless they could prove their spouse was completely dependent upon them. Finally, single female nurses stayed in nurses' quarters, often under the watchful eye of the chief nurse charged with seeing "that the morale of the nurses is kept at a high standard."[56] Women who chose to live off base had to forfeit housing pay. These were not the same standards for men in the army. Male officers could marry, have dependents, and receive dependent pay and allowance for housing. Single men in the army also had the option of staying in single-officers' housing or living off base.[57] In short, army men did not have to endure the same custodial supervision that female nurses suffered.

Female nurses wondered, and rightfully so, whether male nurses would expect the same benefits as other male officers. The overwhelming answer to this question was a devastating yes from military officials and others explaining the likely consequences of male nurse integration. Take, for example, the summary about policies and regulations for male nurses from Lt. Col. Katherine Baltz, assistant to the chief of the ANC:

> Insofar as quarters, dependents, and marriage are concerned, male nurses should be given the same rights and privileges as all other male officers and certainly the handling of marriage should be on exactly the same basis as for other male officers, including eligibility to be commissioned in the Regular Army if the male is married. It is believed that the female nurse will understand completely. . . . It places the responsibility on the women as a mother to keep the home and be with her children, while it is accepted mores that the man be the chief support. Therefore, it is believed that we would be criticized very highly for restricting a group of men from a commission because of marriage.[58]

These likely consequences helped explain, in yet another way, the reluctance to support male nurses in their attempt to integrate the ANC. Further, it highlighted the inequality between female nurse officers and officers in the rest of the army. While the ANC was part of the regular army because of the Army-Navy Nurse Act of 1947, this did not mean that there was complete equity between officers of either sex. Accepted social mores during the postwar period recognized two standards when it came to the benefits and privileges military women could expect, as Baltz acknowledged in her response to the male nurse question. Therefore, female nurses rationalized that male nurse integration brought few benefits to women.

Nursing was one of few occupations where women, of any race, assumed some power over men. Nurse officers often directed enlisted medical personnel that included male medics and orderlies within the hospital environment. It made sense that women were extremely protective of an occupation where gender characteristics allowed them to claim unprecedented autonomy and authority and professional opportunities in civil society and in the service of their country. According to a 1950 Gallup Poll, more than one-third of the women questioned chose nursing as the top profession for women.[59] This provides a sense of how important nursing was for women who wanted a working life outside the home. In protecting their domain, however, some women also supported the continuation of the same gendered system they had fought against in their own struggle for opportunity. Lt. Col. Rosalie D. Colhoun, for example, wrote that "the recent war convinced most doctors, as well as the patients, that the female nurse inspired and contributed comfort and courage, which the male nurse could not give."[60] Lt. Col. Augusta L. Short pointed out that the "male population of the Army are the greatest objectors" because "most psychiatrists prefer the female nurse for psychological reasons" and "any place where a male nurse would be better, we have well-trained enlisted men."[61] Colhoun's and Short's focus on the deficiencies of male nurses and natural abilities of female nurses were not new arguments, and it was these arguments that nursing advocates used to establish the nurse corps as female in 1901. These were also the arguments used to keep men out of the nurse corps during World War II.

Colhoun's and Short's purpose was not just to bolster the position of female nurses but, more important, to keep men out of the nurse corps. They pointed to the fact that men would not work well within this female environment, nor did they really have a right to. Colhoun and Short were not alone in their opinion. "Nursing the sick is definitely a women's prerogative," commented another nurse officer. Maj. Mabel G. Stott was even more pointed on the topic when she questioned the ability of men to take orders from women. "What would be the attitude of male officers serving under the command and leadership of female officers?" Stott concluded by suggesting that "it is not felt that male officers would be satisfied, happy, or co-operative in serving under this authority."[62] Given that male nurses increasingly worked with and under the supervision of female nurses in civilian hospitals, these viewpoints suggest the differences between civil and military nursing.[63] Feeling as though "their" institution were under attack, some female officers suggested that the wider nursing profession did not truly support male nurse integration but was pressured from a small minority to accept the idea. Lieutenant Colonel Short, for example, ended her letter to the chief of the ANC by stating, "Miss Dietrich does not believe that changing the law to include male nurses is the opinion of the ANA but it is because the male Section is bringing pressure on them."[64]

Female nurse officers' recommendations for alternatives to accepting male nurses further revealed their determination to protect their position in the ANC. Many of the suggestions reiterated the gendered nature of the profession and focused on protecting women's position within it. There is a sense among many of the recommendations that nurse officers feared that the addition of men would lead to a loss of authority for women, that having fought hard for recognition and respect, women would ultimately have to defer to men.[65] For example, many of the officers recommended that the chief of the nurse corps should always be female, as should the chief nurses at each hospital and each unit. Lt. Col. Colhoun pointed out that although men "would eventually expect to hold administrative positions, . . . this would be resented by the majority of female nurses."[66] As women made up the majority of the organization and as the duties of chief nurses encompassed much more than nursing, female officers argued that this would be the most practical solution if males joined the nurse corps.[67]

Officers also recommended three options for male acceptance that would keep men as a minority of the organization; these options evoked the suggestions and policies pertaining to black female nurses during World War II. These are important because they attempted to institutionalize men's marginal role in the profession and because they hinted at earlier civil rights concessions meant to sustain the status quo. First, female officers suggested that men be included as reservists, commissioned only in the event of emergencies. This gave men short-term duty tours but no permanent place in the nurse corps. For the professional male nurse, this would mean no job security and showed a distinct lack of respect from the female nurse officers. Second, and even more disconcerting, was the suggestion of a quota system that based the number of males nurses accepted into the nurse corps on the "estimated needs and positions to which male nurses may be assigned to the best advantage."[68] This suggestion—that the U.S. Army set the parameters by which only the smallest percentage of men were used as nurses, even when nursing shortages were great—was profoundly reminiscent of the experiences of African American female nurses earlier in the century. Finally, several of the nurse officers suggested that male nurses receive commission in alternate areas of the Medical Department. They looked to the Medical Allied Science or Sanitary Engineering Sections as places where male nurses could use their training to gain officer status. In these areas, male nurses gained the recognition and status they desperately wanted, but they would not be nurses or members of the ANC.[69]

Nearly eight months after the American Nurses' Association notified the ANC of its intention, Congresswoman Francis Payne Bolton introduced H.R. 9398 in the second session of the Eighty-First Congress. Bolton had unsuccessfully introduced similar legislation on several occasions throughout the 1940s.[70] This new bill, however, had the momentum of the successful Army-Navy Nurse Act of 1947, strong support from national nursing groups, and mounting Cold War tensions. Bolton and the ANA hoped these factors and well-placed campaigning would make the 1950 bill a triumph.[71] H.R. 9398, a bill "to provide for the appointment of male citizens as nurses in the Army, Navy, and Air Force, and for other purposes," went to the Armed Services Committee for review.[72] Initial responses from the military were favorable; as the surgeon general stated that the Department of the Army was not opposed to the enactment of the bill but was studying the subject closely.

Early in the process, it appeared that male nurses would gain acceptance in the ANC without any of the limitations suggested by female nurses. Male nurses cheered what they viewed as the most "progressive action" taken to date on their behalf. Registered nurse Earl McDowell hoped that the passage of Bolton's bill would finally end "sex discrimination," and he pointed out that his experiences and those of other male nurses during World War II proved how invaluable they were in combat areas.[73] With the United States becoming increasingly involved in the hostilities in Korea, the passage of the bill seemed imminent, as by early fall the army was having trouble getting women either to join the ANC or to move to active duty. *RN Magazine*, for example, noted that an "Army appeal for 650 nurses directed chiefly to those in the Reserves . . . [resulted in] only 142 nurses," most of whom were young, new nurses and not those already in the reserves.[74] This was because of the "marriage and dependent" policies in place within the ANC and because of ongoing support for traditional gender roles generated by postwar anxiety.[75] Yet male nurses had only to call attention to the circumstances of women physicians and the army to highlight the contradictory nature of prescribed gender roles.

Throughout 1950 the U.S. Army and Navy also debated about the use and commissioning of women physicians in each military branch. "The fair sex is posing a problem for the Army and Navy who disagree on how women physicians should be commissioned," *RN Magazine* noted in September.[76] Both branches agreed they needed women physicians, but whereas the navy preferred to commission them as WAVES and assign them to duties on that basis, the army supported commissioning female doctors as they did their male counterparts. The bill under consideration, H.R. 4384, would allow the appointment of female doctors to the Army Medical Department on the same basis as men officers. While a sex-based employment policy did not govern the Army Medical Department, the army's support of the bill for female doctors and unenthusiastic response to the commissioning of male nurses appeared inconsistent with the army's attempt to provide adequate medical staff for its soldiers and their families.[77] Beyond the sex of the provider, male nurses argued that there was little difference between commissioning women physicians and men nurses.

By October 1950 the Department of Defense and the army reconsidered their initial favorable attitude toward the new male nurse bill. This was due in part to the information received from the ANC and the Women Medical Specialist Department on the inclusion of male nurses. The Department of Defense reported to Carl Vinson, the chairman of the Committee on

Armed Services, that it opposed the ratification of H.R. 9398. In fact, all three branches of the military rejected the male nurse bill. Although each branch suggested that the major reason behind this decision was the Army-Navy Nurse Act of 1947, equally apparent to most were the continued negative views of men nurses and the championing of nursing as a gender-specific occupation.[78] Military officials argued that the 1947 changes to the Army-Navy Nurse Act succeeded in part because the provisions it gave to nurses assumed that the nurse corps would remain a female-only group. They further argued that those provisions, including rules on marriage, children, and retirement, were inappropriate for male nurse officers because the rules were not in line with the benefits received by other male officers, nor did they align with the advantages traditionally enjoyed by men in civilian society.

The Defense Department also pointed out the same organizational problems noted by female nurse officers. They argued that administration, personnel, and housing became problematic with the inclusion of men, and they feared that the nurse corps would consequentially become ineffective. Interestingly, these were the exact arguments the army used to fight the Fahy Committee concerning the integration of African Americans in accordance with E.O. 9981.[79] Given the military's and Defense Department's focus on future missions and Cold War hostilities, the army felt that the distraction of integrating male nurses was unacceptable. The presumption that male nurses would cause more distraction than good troubled male nurse supporters because they witnessed the integration of women into other areas of the army with simple adjustments to policies. Nevertheless, while the Department of Defense had already made its decision concerning the matter in early October, it gave no public announcement of that opinion, nor did it respond to inquirers about an official decision until late October.[80] This was more than just a ploy to keep the public in the dark; the Department of Defense recognized how sensitive the subject had become among nursing leaders and members of the public. As was the case in the later years of World War II, the Defense Department faced the difficult job of justifying its position to the public while the country entered another conflict.

H.R. 9398 essentially stalled in the Committee on Armed Services in late 1950. The support of several congressional representatives, the American Nurses' Association, and labor organizations such as the American Federation of Government Employees could not save the bill once all three branches of the military had rejected it.[81] Instead, as one nurse corps historian pointed out, the need for nurses "was [again] outweighed by the unfair but even more powerful prejudices against male nurses."[82] Fears about the nation's defenses and the need for national unity went only so far. In 1950, nursing and military service remained tightly bound to traditional gender identities and roles. For their own economic security, female nurse officers helped perpetrate the continuation of these gendered understandings.

The attitude of the army nurse officers and the decision of the Committee on Armed Forces were difficult to understand because they were inconsistent with the civilian nursing profession at mid-century. Nursing organizations focused on integrating men and minority women into the profession as a means of mobilizing nurses for national security. In 1951 the Joint Committee on Nursing in National Security, for example, issued a statement on the policies needed to organize nurses and nursing services during an emergency. These policies were based on a number of general assumptions, according to the joint committee. The first assumption was that the military would make "use of men nurses and auxiliary workers." However, military opinions about male nurses clearly indicated that national security was not the means for integration but was, rather, the reason to maintain the status quo.[83] The result, of course, was that male nurses found themselves in the same position they had been in during World War II, serving in the military without any guarantee of using their skills. Already in November 1950, the American Association of Nurse Anesthetists, for example, noted the drafting of one of the forty-one male nurse members in the army as a private first class.[84]

Korea: Testing Race Desegregation/Debating Gender Roles

While the debate over male nurse inclusion continued within the ranks of the military and among male nurse supporters, pressing hostilities in Korea highlighted a new phase in the Cold War. The involvement of the United States and Soviet Union in a larger conflict led to the escalation and expansion of what was internally a civil war in Korea. Officially known as a "police action," or the Korean War in the United States, the U.S. military found itself fighting a war that was not ever a declared war.[85] The ANC provided care in an environment—both stateside and abroad—unlike any other in its fifty-year history. Estimates vary on the number of ANC nurses who served in Korea over the course of the conflict, but nurse corps numbers during this period fluctuated between thirty-five hundred and five thousand.[86] The army had nurses stationed across the United States, Europe, and areas in East Asia, including Japan and Korea in the first few years of the 1950s.

Hostilities in Korea began on June 25, 1950; in less than two weeks the first twelve Army nurses arrived in Pusan to form the 8055th Mobile Army

Surgical Hospital (MASH).[87] MASH units were the medical units closest to the front that employed army nurses. Throughout the three-year hostilities, army nurses became renowned for their hard work, courage, and devotion to duty, with praise from surgeons and soldiers. This dedication and the Medical Department's advances in combat medicine translated to an astonishing survival rate. The death rate for soldiers admitted to hospitals was reduced from forty for every one thousand patients admitted during World War II to under ten men per one thousand admitted to army hospitals during the Korean War.[88] These accomplishments did not make the ANC or its members immune, however, to social struggles in the United States. This was the military's first opportunity to test the grand experiment of an desegregated Army. It was also an opportunity to test and continue the debate about gender roles in the ANC as both nursing shortages generally, and combat conditions specifically, pushed many to reassess the nurse corps' insistence on a single-sexed organization.[89]

Civil rights activists paid particular attention to the activities of African Americans serving with the armed forces following the passage of Executive Order 9981. The Korean War and the military's activities in other overseas regions provided the perfect opportunities to observe the effectiveness of integration. As they had done during World War II, the black press played the role of watchdog and cheerleader, celebrating the activities of black soldiers—men and women—who served overseas, and reporting any violations of the president's order. Littered throughout the pages of the *Chicago Defender*, *Pittsburgh Courier*, and *Baltimore Afro-American* were reports of equal rights successes and failures that revealed contradictions to the integration of the armed forces. Four years after the passage of E.O. 9981, for example, the *Chicago Defender* praised the reversal of the navy's exclusion of African American women the year before the Korean War began. In contrast, the *Baltimore Afro-American* reported a commanding officer's admission that segregated army units were stationed at some European bases.[90]

The complicated nature of integration was even more apparent in Korea. Racism and segregation, employment opportunities and the pressures of war collided. Just as the black unemployment rate rose in the United States following World War II, so too did the rates of black enlistments. And yet segregation among troops remained the de facto procedure. Army officials continued to argue that segregation was a "national defense imperative," especially as integration highlighted racism and prejudice among white and black troops and among the enlisted and officer corps. Bound to the African American reaction to the war was a community responding to the uneven commitment to integration by the army, the debate over the place of African Americans in a war against other "colored" people, and the acceleration of the domestic civil rights movement. The press, both black and white, captured the complexity and tension of integration beautifully. Early in the war the press lauded African American soldiers for their bravery in one of the first major victories for the U.S. and U.N. forces; yet by early 1951 the court-martial of thirty-nine black soldiers charged with insubordination overshadowed the early successes of black soldiers. It led to a sustained scrutiny of black participation in Korea—as suspect from the white press, and as another space in which civil rights activists needed to watch in the black press.[91]

The role of racial publicity had repercussions both domestically and internationally for the United States. Within the framework of Cold War politics, the United States used the American military not only to defend but also to advance the nation's dedication to freedom, liberty, and equality.[92] In failing to reconcile American principles with American practices even in its military, the United States risked, according to the president of the National Council of Negro Women, "betraying the hopes of mankind."[93] How could the United States complete its Cold War mission with such egregious displays of its own halfhearted support of equality? Truman's nondiscrimination policy went only so far in demonstrating the best of life in a democratic society. The failure to portray even a unified military to the rest of the world proved that the nation's social problems were not resolved as the result of public policy.[94]

The experience of African American nurses exemplifies the contradiction between military policy and individual social beliefs and attitudes concerning race relations in the postwar period. Captain Margaret Bailey remembered her integration experience as a challenge to President Truman's decree. Three years after the passage of E.O. 9981, Bailey and two other nurses arrived at the 98th General Hospital in Munich, Germany. They were the first black officers stationed at the hospital and the first black female officers in the area, but they had every expectation of living with the other nursing staff. To the dismay and disappointment of Bailey, they lived not with the other nurses at the hospital but in a separate house away from the hospital. This was a "setback in integration," and while Bailey admitted that most of the staff and residents near the hospital became accustomed to and welcomed the presence of the black nurses, she and the other black nurses still dealt with individual cases of discrimination and racism.[95] Bailey also remembered one incident that involved her dismissal by a doctor at the hospital. Although hurt by his actions, Bailey stated she had to make "a mental adjustment in order to be effective" in her work.[96] That Bailey and other African Americans had to adjust their thinking on integration for the greater good reveals the tenuous prospect of complete desegregation of minorities in the armed forces. The practice of nondiscrimination was a compromise and the fulfillment of a need that did not necessarily change the beliefs or behaviors of individuals.

According to the official Army Nurse Corps history, "only a few problems arose in connection with the integration effort in the combat setting of Korea."[97] One chief nurse noted the inevitable situation of either a white or a black nurse serving as a minority among the majority of the opposite race. In this situation, the nurse noted, "conversations, interests, and customs, were so different" that both would be embarrassed and uncomfortable. This, she said, indirectly affected the performance and nursing care provided in that situation.[98] Underlining these comments was the sense that for some, race was both an acceptable and a natural way to organize society and the workplace. The military had publically proclaimed since World War II that the military was not the place to test and change social relations. Nevertheless, the armed forces found themselves caught between the president's and federal government's attempts to rally the nation around the principles of American democracy and freedom and the reality of social relationships in the United States.[99] Non-discrimination and thus integration constituted an artificial directive imposed on the armed forces by the president without thought to the reality of personal beliefs and customs. This was especially true on the home front, where local customs distorted the possible benefits of E.O. 9981.

The U.S. military played a central role in promoting an image of the United States that was in stark opposition to the Soviet Union. In some ways, this was easier to do at stations and bases outside the United States, although not always, as the experience of Margaret Bailey proved. According to Brig. Gen. Lillian Dunlap, the difficulty of promoting integration and unity really became a chronicle of life on and off base in the United States. Stationed both stateside and abroad between World War II and 1975, Dunlap noted that in the early years of integration of the military, difficulties emerged, especially on bases located in the south and southwest. On base, Dunlap said, "we all lived in the nurses' quarters. They were accepted . . . but then, when we went off post it was a rude awakening to us—the whites—that we couldn't go into the restaurants together. Or we couldn't go shopping together."[100] Set against the backdrop of an expanding civil rights movement, the race problems in the U.S. military and ANC serve as a constant reminder that American society was in a state of social flux in the postwar period. Tightly bound cultural beliefs were tested and challenged. The reality was that in the wake of a depression, a World War, and a global Cold War, the racial status quo and, as we shall see, strictly defined gender roles were genuinely difficult to maintain.[101]

As far as some members of the public and military were concerned, combat during the Korean War era made the subject of integration and nursing about more than racial integration in the ANC. The long-debated question of male nurses continued after the 1950 and 1951 legislative attempt by Congresswoman Bolton and the ANA stalled in the Armed Services Committee. Supporters of the bill and of expanded opportunities for women in the military believed that beyond ensuring a unified military through integration, the defense of the country also meant reevaluating how gender shaped opportunities in the United States military. In the ANC, this included reassessing the placement of female nurses near combat. For example, while the chief of the Army Nurse Corps' Far East Command commended the job of her nurses in the Far East, she reminded newspaper readers that "in oriental warfare, women nurses have no place near the battlefront . . . bitter experiences prove the enemy ruthless and unprincipled—we know too well what would happen if nurses were captured."[102] Her opinion that army nurses were in essence "a distinct liability and hazard to themselves and the troops" was just the sort of information that male nurse supporters needed to continue pressing their own cause.[103] Historically, the ANC and military had been able to reassure those who worried about women's proximity to combat by guaranteeing that nurses were well behind front lines and protected. Nevertheless, the capture of nurses in the South Pacific during World War II shattered this imagined safety net.[104] These circumstances tested the conventional and traditional understanding that nursing was best suited to the females of the population, as it suggested the confinement of women to only the strictest and most protected locations.

The idea of using male medics in combat-forward MASH units gained some credence during the Korean War, although the army remained adamant about the integration of male nurses in the ANC. In late September 1952 army surgeon Melvin Horwitz wrote to his wife about his transfer to the 8225th MASH unit. In his letters, we find out that the army decided to reactivate the 8225th as an experiment to test the possibility of nurseless hospitals, using corpsmen in their place.[105] The experiment, Dr. Horwitz later learned, was the result of a larger plan by the army to attempt an amphibious assault off the east coast of Korea behind Chinese lines.[106] Had the plan moved forward, this would have made the 8225th the hospital farthest north and closest to combat. In this situation, it appears that the army had heeded the concerns about women debated in the national press, especially nurses near the battlefront. This decision also revealed the army's willingness to consider having men serve in nursing positions, although not as nurses.

The army abandoned the proposal of an amphibious assault within a month of the 8225th reactivation, but the experiment of the "corpsmen nurse" remained. Throughout the fall of 1952 and winter of 1953 Dr. Horwitz's letters present a particularly interesting view into how the lack of female nurses affected the running of a MASH unit. His observations reveal two distinct concerns about a hospital without female nurses. The first was a morale factor, as Dr. Horwitz writes that "most of them [men], including doctors, lament the fact that there will be no nurses at this MASH. . . . I need no nurses to provide female company."[107] Two nurses did accompany the 8225th to train the corpsmen; Horwitz's statement implies, however, that many of the men were concerned about the serious lack of female companionship. In fact, his comments suggest that for a number of men, nurses had a double role in this environment. Professionally, nurses were caregivers; privately, they served as companions, supporters, and morale boosters for men. This was neither the first nor the last time that the duty or obligation of female nurses was conceived within the framework of morale; the presence of American women, particularly nurses, was often remembered as one of the best morale boosters for soldiers away from home. Nevertheless, the doctor's remark reveals one of the complicated reasons for the general reluctance and opposition to male nurses.

The second concern about using corpsmen instead of female nurses was their lack of training and professionalism. Throughout a five-month period, Dr. Horwitz routinely complained to his wife about the laziness of the corpsmen, the need to supervise them, which burdened others with more work, and his growing alarm about patient care because of their lack of training. "A corpsman who didn't know any better took an oral temperature. . . . I hope it won't be necessary for someone to die because of a mistake before they send them [the nurses] to us. The boys just haven't had the experience with patients."[108] Nearing the end of five months without a full female nursing staff, Horwitz writes, "It has been shown that our corpsmen cannot take care of the [patients] properly in post-op." He continues, "At the meeting, we all told the Col., in turn, that the patients were being endangered by lack of good nursing care."[109] It was not until the end of February 1953 that the doctor writes with relief, "We are being assigned 5 nurses. The experiment is over. They have decided they cannot run a MASH without trained personnel."[110] While Horwitz focused on the training differences between nurses and corpsmen, he made no suggestion of commissioning male nurses as a possible substitute for female nurses in combat-forward areas. The discussion about the integration of male nurses was ongoing within the military, the civilian nursing establishment, and the federal government, and yet the failure of the doctor to mention even cursorily the use of male nurses suggests a disconnect between the medical establishment and nursing personnel debates. It is also an indication of just how much the nursing profession remained tightly bound to women and gender roles in the postwar period.

In the United States, male nurses and their supporters bemoaned what they viewed as a double standard employed by the military. By mid-1952, the army as well as the other branches of the military accepted female physicians in both their reserve corps and as part of the regular military. Registered nurse Morris Wolf reminded readers that the U.S. Armed Services "have recognized the existence and professional equality of women physicians by granting them officers' rank and status."[111] In other words, the military eventually resolved many of the arguments about legal barriers and administrative problems associated with the integration of female physicians into male-dominated medical areas.[112] So, what was different about male nurses? Did, as Wolf asked, the "sex of the practitioner matter?"[113]

Certainly, this was the question that male nurses and their supporters repeatedly asked throughout their campaign and pointedly answered in the negative. An even more important point, however, is that the failure to integrate male nurses highlighted an underlying fear by female nurses about the loss of authority and dominance in a profession they had come to control. Additionally, male nurse integration also fostered anxiety about the distortion of gender roles and exposed gender inequalities most often experienced by women in the workplace. As African American female nurses had before them, male nurses wanted acceptance and recognition based on their professional training, not some biological factor they could not change. Nevertheless, attached to American understandings of biological and racial difference was access to or denial of economic opportunities and benefits. Female nurses worried that male nurse demand for acceptance as nurse officers meant that male nurses *expected* the same benefits afforded other male military officers.[114] This would mean that male nurses gained benefits in the ANC not available to female nurses, creating an environment of inequality and resentment within the nurse corps.

Male nurse advocates changed tactics in their integration campaign following the negative reports from the Department of Defense in late 1950. Frances Bolton suggested two ways of commissioning male nurses during the Korean War. The first was an option that several female nurse officers proffered in early 1950. Bolton suggested to the chairperson of the Armed Services Committee that he consider male nurses for the position of medical assistants. The medical assistant was an officer who served as the adminis-trative assistant to the medical officer. The position required the person to have a medical background, as the assistant often helped the medical officer in emergencies. Bolton believed that such a position would be fitting of the skills and training of male nurses, and as an added bonus medical assistants could serve as assistant battalion surgeons at aid stations near front lines.[115] This would solve the dilemma of placing female nurses near combat while at the same time relieve fears about territorial overlap with female nurses. Furthermore, it would guarantee that the Army had a viable alternative to using underqualified men with little more than six-weeks' training, as the experiment with "corpsmen nurses" at the MASH 8225th later revealed.[116] Ultimately, Bolton's change in strategy reflected an acknowledgement that the greatest obstacle to male nurse integration remained the fact that in the eyes of many, male nurses were the wrong sex for caregiving.[117]

Unlike African American female nurses who could and did argue that re-gardless of race, their sex and the gender characteristics assigned to it made them caregivers, male nurses, hindered by gender conventions, continued to face the implication of being effeminate, "crooked," or unseemly. Men nurses did point to the historic connection between manhood and military participation, but the military, the extreme representation of societal beliefs and values, remained firmly entrenched in the perception of the "fiction of the woman's touch," as one male registered nurse labeled it.[118] High-ranking military officers perpetuated this stereotype. One medical officer remarked to the chief of the ANC, "When I get sick, I want a nurse that will bring a women's touch, and if it is a male nurse that brings a women's touch, I don't want him."[119] A former chief of the nurse corps also remembered comments such as "look at the femininity" in reference to male nurses.[120] The sense that something was "wrong" with male nurses was alive and well and underlined the pervasive anxiety about homosexuality in the military and civilian society. This was especially true in the postwar period, where charges of homosexual behavior became linked to threats to the nation's security and family life.[121] The military, like many in civilian society, feared that male nurses were in fact sexual deviants propagating taboo behavior. Bolton clearly understood this when she suggested her compromise to commissioning male nurses to Chairman Vinson.

> I am aware of the thought in the minds of many high officials that male nurses exhibit a high incidence of homosexuality, and that this would be a tragic thing for the Armed Forces. Actually . . . the incidence of sexual devi-ants among this group was no higher, was lower in fact, than among other

groups . . . The charge is certainly unfair to the overwhelming percentage of well adjusted normal healthy male nurses.[122]

In emphasizing the "normality" of male nurses and, earlier in the letter, the suggestion to use male nurses as medical assistants, Bolton hoped to get men commissioned in a way that made everyone comfortable with their presence. In other words, as the specific gendered behaviors attached to the definition of nurses made men's role in this profession suspicious, Bolton hoped that renaming their duties would lead to officer's commission. Bolton introduced no bill to support this suggestion, however, and male nurses who attempted to gain commissions through the Medical Service Corps failed.[123] Bolton's only option was to reintroduce the bill to commission men in the ANC.

Bolton's second strategy for the appointment of male nurses into the ANC shifted the focus away from the regular army to the reserve corps. As with her suggestion to commission male nurses as medical assistants, Bolton viewed the reserve corps as a preliminary step in gaining recognition for male nurses in the military. This ploy worked in commissioning the first female physician officers, and she hoped it would work in male nurses' favor.[124] In early 1954 Bolton addressed the House of Representatives to introduce the bill that would authorize the appointment of male nurses as reserve officers. Unlike previous attempts, the new bill had some support from the Department of Defense because it did not reflect a mandatory change. Instead, the bill allowed each branch of the military either to decline instituting the change or to employ the new law to bolster their numbers in times of peace and war. Bolton and male nurse leader LeRoy Craig pointed out that the passage of such a bill would help increase the supply of nurses to the armed forces, especially during emergencies. It would also reduce the drain on civilian nursing, and help increase the number of men interested and enrolling in nursing schools.[125] In light of the recent hostilities in Korea and the shortages of nurses in civil hospitals and in the military, proponents believed that appointing male nurses in the reserve corps was the best and most forward-thinking move the armed forces could take. Interestingly, events taking place outside the military and the United States helped further strengthen support for the bill.

In the spring of 1954 the defeat of the French at Dien Bien Phu provided additional support for the argument in favor of male nurses.[126] Among those who faced the horrifying events that unfolded at the fortress between March and May was a stranded female nurse assigned to an airborne unit. The experiences of this nurse, later known as the "Angel of Dien Bien Phu," represented to Bolton and others the single most important reason for training and accepting male nurses, the possibility of placing women's lives in jeopardy near combat. Even as the role of women in the military evolved since World War II, public discourse remained adamant that women be as protected as possible from the dangers of combat. Attempts to address the safety of nurses in combat areas were recurring, but the gendered nature of nursing work and concerns about the training of men nurses consistently trumped these worries. Bolton saw the Dien Bien Phu incident as a needed dose of reality for those who still argued against the addition of male nurses. After all, the army was lucky to have avoided similar circumstances in Korea, but this might not be the case in the future. No "young women of 29 [should] witness the tragedy of the wounded of Dien Bien Phu," Bolton reminded Congress. Instead, in times of war, male nurse reserve officers could be called upon to "apply their training in areas where we should never ask a woman to serve."[127] In short, Bolton relied on the old argument that the defense of the nation and protection of female nurses demanded the addition of male nurses. This was one argument that male nurses and supporters had promoted since World War II, although with little success.

In the summer of 1955 several merging factors succeeded in finally getting the bill passed by Congress: the continuing difficulty of recruiting women nurses into the armed forces during the postwar period, the backing of professional nursing organizations, and the support of individual nursing activists. These factors, however, were not the sole reasons the Bolton Bill of 1955, H.R. 2559, finally passed and was signed into law during that summer.[128] Instead, these factors, coupled with the exploitation of Cold War fears and events during the postwar period, ended the remaining barriers against male nurse inclusion in the ANC. This was not, however, the end to prejudice against them. Male nurses remained suspect to many, but Bolton, LeRoy Craig, and others could and did emphasize nursing shortages, strong beliefs that women should never face combat, and Cold War tensions to negotiate men into the ANC.[129] Edward L. T. Lyon became the first man to receive a commission in the ANC, when he entered active duty on October 10, 1955.

Bolton also connected the male nurse question to a larger debate and fight over discrimination and equal rights taking place in the United States. She viewed the passage of what she later identified as "my equal rights for men bill" in much the same way she viewed the end to barriers for African American female nurses a decade early. In fact, she understood discrimination against male nurses as one more case of inequality in the profession that had to be remedied for the health of the entire country. By recognizing the legitimate place of male nurses in the armed forces, the legislation helped end discrimination in the occupation as a whole. Bolton viewed the male nurse situation as an unusual example of "the normal problem of discrimination between men and women in the occupations," but a case of discrimination nevertheless.[130] She focused on the fact that there was a place and need for every qualified trained nurse within the nursing profession; out-of-date beliefs on racial aptitude and gender capabilities had no role in the modern profession.

Civil rights activists could argue that the same could be said of modern society in general. Bolton may not have originally understood it that way, but many viewed her work in the nursing field as a larger commentary for improving economic and social equality in American society. At a commencement talk to a group of African American nurses, Bolton pointed out to the young women that their contributions to society were not limited to nursing. They made a great contribution to the "field of race relations" as well. Their mission was to play a role in the "growth of tolerance and understanding." At the same time, responding to Bolton's view on gender equality, one reader said, "She is probably right. . . . If we're going to have equality of the sexes, it must work both ways."[131]

Ten years after the end of World War II, efforts to defend the nation and promote its democratic tenets met a society in social flux. Long-held beliefs about race relations, gender roles, and even equal rights faced new challenges domestically and internationally. The growing civil rights movement accomplished unparalleled success by achieving both support and prudence in the face of Cold War tensions. Yet the push for stability following World War II also meant a strong pull for returning to and embracing traditional values and beliefs. Truman's policy of nondiscrimination in the armed forces as a means to strengthen the U.S. image abroad and reduce domestic civil rights tensions had mixed results as neither a complete failure nor a complete success. The ANC experience during this period exemplified this contradiction. It revealed the tenuous nature of integration as the pathway to social and economic equality.

5

The Quality of a Person

Race and Gender Roles Re-Imagined?

With the acceptance of male nurses in 1955, the Army Nurse Corps found itself in the unusual position of appearing to be a vanguard in the fight for an even greater conception of civil rights. Over the next ten years the ANC struggled with the far-reaching ramifications of this decision on everything from day-to-day operations, wages, and benefits, to a fundamental redefinition of the role of nursing within the army. Throughout the period between the mid-1950s and the late 1960s, the ANC and its members simultaneously endorsed and impeded attempts to restructure race and gender roles and standards while endeavoring to meet the practical nursing needs of the U.S. Army.[1] At the advent of the Vietnam War, following the passage of the Civil Rights Act of 1964, the ANC represented a new frontier of integration in the labor force. Yet the reality of the situation proved more complex. This chapter examines how integration issues within the ANC reflected the complicated nature of a broader domestic civil rights struggle.

In the period between the end of the Korean War and overt U.S. participation in Vietnam, national conversations around civil rights expanded beyond questions of race. With the initial successes of the post–World War II civil rights movement, exemplified by the passage of Executive Order 9981 and *Brown v. Board of Education*, it was clear that there was room for more groups under the tent of social justice. The nation grappled with questions about gender roles and sexual equality, continuing the focus on social and economic inequality through new lenses. Several different groups began to champion the idea that it was the quality of the person, not their race, sex, religion, or ethnicity that should determine their place in society. Though not a single movement, this turbulent period united individuals and groups through the promotion of political change and social justice activities as a means of ensuring a more inclusive citizenry. Against this backdrop, the military was not engaged in active battle, but there was certainly no elimination of Cold War tensions. There was continued pressure to remain on high alert and at full readiness. In this setting, the military's focus on organizational mandates, driven by pragmatic needs such as ongoing nursing shortages, forced a restructuring far more progressive than the organization or the individuals involved were perhaps prepared for.

In civil society, and as it had in the previous ten years, the nursing profession at large continued to position itself as one of several professions whose obligation it was to provide leadership in the efforts to promote broader definitions of equality. This contrasts directly with the army, including the ANC, which continued to proclaim that the military was not an "instrument of social reform."[2] Ironically, of course, the army's actions, viewed within the context of domestic civil rights activities, contradicted this assertion and ultimately advanced integration more than any other single organization in the country.

Military Civil Rights

The 1954 *Brown* decision ushered in the classical phase of the civil rights movement. It overturned the historic 1896 Supreme Court decision in *Plessy v. Ferguson* that sanctioned "separate but equal." While civil rights activities over the next decade eventually broke down the entire structure of Jim Crow laws that had emerged and expanded at the turn of the nineteenth century, they also gave rise to a growing movement of conservative whites *resisting* civil rights activities and goals. Some opponents of civil rights goals denounced the 1954 *Brown* decision as inspired by Communism; even the U.S. Army was not immune to charges and fears of communist infiltration.[3] Historians have argued that anticommunism narrowed the goals of social justice movements in the postwar period as a whole.[4] Conservative whites used anticommunist rhetoric to fend off social change by highlighting a traditional American ethos of limited government and economic independence. They formed White Citizens' Councils to intimidate those who challenged segregation and discrimination. By the late 1950s, these groups slowed the progress made by civil rights activists and created an environment that was increasingly hostile to initiatives that many conservatives viewed as the invasion of the federal government into state and local matters.[5] They viewed social justice activists as "un-American" and labeled their activities as unpatriotic.[6] This restricted civil rights discourse by limiting the more diverse and radical voices for social change that were the hallmarks of the New Deal period.[7] Yet by emphasizing "the promise of equality," economic opportunity, and access to the rewards of citizenship, civil rights activists argued that they helped strengthen American democracy, not undermine it.[8] They called attention to the ways communists used examples of racial injustice and discrimination in their anti-American propaganda. In this way, civil rights activists could and did cast antidiscrimination as patriotic. Still, the tensions between opposing responses to civil rights objectives proved a challenge for the military.

A socially conservative organization at its root, the military of the United States found it difficult to ignore or resist the changing nature of race relations during the 1950s and early 1960s. Certainly, the military's strict adherence to and reliance on military codes of conduct meant that it was somewhat more manageable for the army to implement changes concerning race and gender norms. Yet the passage of legislation, policies, and directives that focused on the "equality of treatment and opportunity" for men and women in the service, regardless of race, proved as difficult to enforce in the military as it was in civilian society. Inadequate supervision and communication, and an unwillingness of some personnel to support military policies regarding discrimination by setting aside their own personal beliefs, hampered the push for equality. This meant that while the military unintentionally projected an image of leading the charge for social change in American society, especially to the world at large, efforts within the military were more representative of the complicated nature of social reorganization.[9]

Even before World War II, civil rights activists used the United States military as a space to measure the real and symbolic successes of the civil rights movement.[10] In military service, many saw the most obvious place to argue for equality as President Franklin Roosevelt, for example, bound wartime rhetoric to the language of democracy during World War II. Military participation and acceptance of racial minorities, activists hoped, would break down discrimination and translate into better opportunities in civilian society. The passage of Executive Order 9981 and the continuing push to ensure nondiscrimination in the army during the Korean conflict suggested that military integration was moving in the right direction in providing African Americans with better opportunities.

By 1954 the army fulfilled most of the requirements for integration. African Americans had access to better opportunities and leadership roles within the military. These changes extended beyond African Americans to include women and other minorities as well. According to a 1990s study on racial politics and integration in the military during the 1950s, the public and military generally relaxed their focus on race relations in the military after 1954.[11] The integration of the military appeared a success in the opinion of many, and desegregation seemed to resolve racial discrimination on the surface. Yet because of this, civil rights activists wondered whether the U.S. military should take a more active role in civil rights efforts outside the armed forces. The military balked at the idea that it should have any direct participation in domestic civil rights activities, however.[12]

Although the U.S. military tried to distance itself from civilian civil rights struggles, it was not immune to them. Almost nothing shielded military personnel from discriminatory beliefs and treatment beyond military bases. For some, the military's refusal to "exert its influence to advance racial equality beyond its own facilities" signaled a continued adherence to a conservative insistence on staying "neutral in civilian politics." Nevertheless, while military policy with respect to race relations regulated, as one scholar suggested, the behavior of its military personnel, it could not change the "underlying attitudes of them."[13] This fact alone meant that racial tensions continued to exist within and in relation to the United States military. Civilian–military relations in communities that had large populations of military personnel best exemplified this.

Throughout the late 1950s, African American service members objected to discrepancies between their treatment on base and off base. Chapter 4 highlighted some of the realities for nurses stationed at United States military bases in the American South and at installations abroad. African American nurses reported dealing with racist attitudes and behaviors in surrounding communities from Texas to Germany.[14] Race equality policies may have provided black Americans with better opportunities within the military, but they did little to change the treatment and lives of black Americans beyond military boundaries. In much the same way that civil rights advocates argued for the end to race discrimination within the military, they began to argue after 1954 that the military had some responsibility to force an end to race discrimination within the communities serving and surrounding military installations. African American nurse Col. Margaret Bailey remembered it as dealing with the old problem, "No blacks allowed here."[15] Off-base race relations, these advocates contended, played a significant role in the "military readiness and morale" of its service members.[16] Ignoring this role could and did have a detrimental effect on military effectiveness when black families had to live in substandard housing and at great distances from bases. In one startling example, black service members, required by their duties to live in close proximity to an air-defense missile base, nevertheless had to attain special waivers because there were no housing options for African Americans close to the base.[17] The military remained reluctant to get involved with racial affairs in local communities even when faced with overt examples of local race policies affecting military preparedness. Many commanding officers believed these circumstances were civilian matters, closely tied to local custom, and therefore Executive Order 9981 did not apply off base.

In the aftermath of *Brown*, the military had cause to negotiate its response and actions in civilian society. Given the white backlash to military desegregation and other civil rights activities in the late 1950s, the military believed that any action on its part might further incite tensions and debates about the role of the federal government in local communities. Restricting its involvement to military matters guaranteed no divided loyalties and ensured a uniform fighting force amid Cold War fears. Therefore, although the desegregation of the military placed the armed forces in a position of "being ahead of public opinion on a controversial social issue," its actions during the late 1950s were best characterized by ongoing complacency.[18]

The 1960 election of John F. Kennedy did not automatically signal the momentous social changes that would coalesce in American society over the course of the decade. Civil rights reform was not "a high priority for the new president as he entered office."[19] This included both racial civil rights reforms and women and gender rights reforms that reemerged with stunning strength during the 1960s. Instead, Kennedy's priorities remained where they had been during his tenure in Congress, with foreign affairs. Yet Kennedy's interest in such places as Africa helped inform him of the already strong and important connection between the domestic civil rights struggle and foreign relations. Kennedy's inaugural address, in which he observed his victory as a "celebration of freedom" and called on support for human rights at home and abroad, could only hint at the unexpected changes in the social relations of domestic society.[20] Beyond the already tense racial situation, civil rights had come to encapsulate a broader struggle for social, economic, racial, and gender equality in American society.[21]

Between 1960 and 1963, racial civil rights activities entered a period of unparalleled development. Historians often refer to this period as the "movement at high tide." Beginning with the sit-in at Greensboro, North Carolina, in 1960 through the violence of Birmingham, Alabama, and the massive rally in Washington, D.C., in 1963, civil rights participants brought America face to face with injustice and discrimination. National and international media outlets broadcast violent clashes between peaceful demonstrators and white civic authorities on a daily basis. These images, as well as the persistence of civil rights activists, challenged the president and Congress to take action on behalf of all African Americans in the United States.[22]

By the early 1960s the military's reluctance to involve themselves in civilian civil rights issues met with a resurgence of civil rights activism and a new administration willing to use not only the military but also other federal agencies to alleviate discrimination against black Americans. Between 1961 and 1963, the Department of Defense (DOD) issued several regulations that aimed at extending military policies on race discrimination to communities with ties to or located near military installations. This was a complete reversal from their early position of neutrality toward civilian politics. The enforcement of these policies, however, was difficult, given a lack of oversight, internal communication problems, and even an unwillingness of some officers to implement the directives with any regularity.[23] This left many civil rights activists once again dissatisfied with the military's failure to take a decisive stance on race discrimination. To address this situation, the Department of Defense issued Directive 5120.36 in July 1963.

This bold attempt by the DOD held military commanders responsible for enforcing equal rights on and off base. It stated, "Every military commander . . . has the responsibility to oppose discriminatory practices affecting his men and their dependents and to foster equal opportunity for them, not only in areas under his immediate control, but also in nearby communities where they may gather in off-duty hours."[24] In a stunning move that was not lost on either civilian or military officials and that immediately produced criticism from both, the Department of Defense essentially gave military commanders the license to play a role in ending race discrimination in public accommodations even before such actions were declared illegal by the federal government.[25] For an institution that adamantly proclaimed its neutrality when questioned about its role in civil rights, this move was yet one more instance of contradictory behavior. If placed into the context of military preparedness, however, the Department of Defense's directive fits well with past military justifications for bending the boundaries of social custom. Regardless, the DOD's directive had no clear method of implementation or evaluation, which meant that each branch of the military interpreted the directive in its own way. This was a great relief to those who worried about the directive's negative effect on the prospect of a civil rights bill under discussion within the Kennedy-Johnson administration in mid-1963. The directive's lack of coherence stymied it from having a larger role in resolving racial discrimination outside the context of the military base.

THE QUALITY OF A PERSON · 113

The military and Department of Defense's seemingly direct but effectively roundabout participation in the civil rights movement was interesting, given their general policy against individual participation of service members in civil rights protest and activism. Military officials suggested that their policies against individual involvement in civil rights stemmed from a fear that any overt participation in civil rights protest would provoke retaliation against African American service members.[26] This did not stop service members from taking part in protests. While a private in the Women's Army Corps Reserve and a student at North Carolina A&T in the Army Student Nurse Program, Clara Adams-Ender participated in the 1960 sit-ins at the Woolworth's lunch counter in downtown Greensboro, North Carolina. She writes of her participation as one of her "proudest accomplishments" yet gives no indication that she participated in Greensboro in uniform; her status as a reservist as well as military policies against participation in such activities may explain this.[27] It would also help to insulate her personal activities from charges of "representing" the U.S. Army. As a conservative organization, the military functioned well within the inherent social hierarchy of American society; any changes to the hierarchy upset the military as it did civilian society.

The U.S. military also worried that civil rights participation would disrupt the seemingly successful workings of integration within the military. As civil rights protests became more active and dangerous in the first few years of the 1960s, the U.S. military became stricter in its allowances of service members' activities in relation to social justice. In 1963 the relaxation of the policy against individual participation in civil rights protests by an Air Force commander proved just how closely outside observers scrutinized this matter. Two black soldiers gained permission to take part in a civil rights march; when this information became public, the Department of Defense scolded the soldiers' commanding officer and firmly told all commanding officers that this was not acceptable.[28]

The participation of military personnel in civil rights activities was not always so contentious. During World War II, African American service members had lobbied for military desegregation as part of a larger civil rights agenda. These service members worked to exploit the exigencies of wartime to promote the racial integration of the military. This was particularly true of African American female nurses who aimed to integrate the ANC during World War II. Their status as caregivers placed a sympathetic face on civil rights that guaranteed that civil rights leaders took a keen interest in using them to further the movement as a whole. African American female nurse leaders cultivated close ties with almost every prominent civil rights organization, participated in national political strategy meetings, and even had the support of First Lady Eleanor Roosevelt.[29] When the war ended and integration in the ANC was achieved, African American female nurses used their earlier experience to shift the terms of the ongoing debate about the merits of racial integration from quotas to ending the inequality faced by all female nurses.

The integration of the ANC and the dissolution of the National Association of Colored Graduate Nurses (NACGN) in 1950 represented the barriers African American nurses had breached since World War II. While the need for integration had collapsed as a result, the search for full equality in the nursing profession shifted the focus to the fair and equal treatment of black female nurses. Reassurance of either was impossible, but the personal accounts of several black nurses serving in the ANC after 1955 reveal that many were not afraid to speak up when they believed they faced racism. In their memoirs, nurses Col. Margaret Bailey and Brig. Gen. Clara Adams-Ender discuss confronting racism and discrimination in and out of the ranks of the Army Nurse Corps during the 1960s.[30] Their experiences highlighted the reasons that the American Nurses' Association and civilian nursing profession focused their resources and programs on ensuring the fair and equal treatment for nurses of all races and both sexes.

With the simultaneous passage of the 1964 Civil Rights Act, a persistent nurse shortage, and U.S. participation in the Vietnam War, an equality measured not simply by numbers in the nursing profession and the ANC came closer to reality. In the year before his death, President Kennedy moved quietly closer to aiding the cause of civil rights. In late 1962 he issued Executive Order 11063, which prohibited racial and ethnic discrimination in federally owned or supported housing.[31] In the summer of 1963, after peaceful protests turned violent in Birmingham, Alabama, Kennedy introduced a civil rights bill to Congress. Although initially blocked in Congress, following Kennedy's assassination in November 1963, President Johnson announced his plans to support the passage of the civil rights bill. The Civil Rights Act of 1964 was the culmination of a long-fought battle for racial equality; it banned discrimination in public accommodations, which signaled the legal end to racial segregation. It also banned discrimination by employers based on race, color, religion, national origin, and sex.[32] Civil rights activists, who had long voiced that an end to workplace discrimination and fair access to work was the foundation for successful equality, heralded Title VII of the Civil Rights Act as a triumph.

Meant to derail the passage of the Civil Rights Act, the addition of the word "sex" to Title VII spoke to a growing women's rights movement in the early 1960s. Although founded within the context of economic equality between the sexes, by the mid-1960s the women's rights movement pushed a generation of women to challenge the relationships between men and women and between women and the state. Pressures for women to adhere to strictly delineated gender roles in the 1950s occurred at the same time a growing number of Americans acknowledged the necessity of women working outside the home. In 1951, for example, the American Council on Education sponsored a two-day Conference on Women in the Defense Decade. Though framed within the mission of supporting national security, conference goers acknowledged that the pressing need was to ensure fair treatment in the labor force: "[Women] need equal pay for equal work."[33] Ten years later, in 1961, President Kennedy established the President's Commission on the Status of Women.

One of the main purposes of the commission was to examine the status of women, especially as it pertained to discrimination in the workforce. Until her death in 1962, Eleanor Roosevelt led the commission in exploring issues relating to American women. While not attempting to promote full equality between the sexes, the commission was the president's attempt to balance the demand for traditional female protection with those who wished to promote an Equal Rights Amendment (ERA). More important, however, it signaled renewed attention to equality among the sexes. The commission's report, published two years later, laid the foundation for the passage of the Equal Pay Act of 1963.[34] In the declaration of purpose during the congressional hearings, the U.S. Senate stated that it denounced sex discrimination for a number of reasons, including: sex discrimination "depresses wage and living standard for employees necessary for their health and efficiency," and "it prevents the maximum utilization of the available labor resources."[35] These reasons had long been arguments both civilian and military nurses used to address personnel shortages and inequality between male and female nurses.

Nursing Civil Rights

Since the founding of the Intergroup Relations Committee, the American Nurses' Association pushed the profession and those interested in nursing to support civil rights issues introduced in Congress.[36] By the mid-1950s the association's policies firmly established its commitment to racial and gender equality, at least among nursing leaders. For example, as part of the bylaws on intergroup relations, the organization stated that they would appoint individuals to their staff and committees and would offer registration, counseling, and job placement "without discrimination as to race, creed, color, or sex." Furthermore, the association developed an Economic Security Program that concentrated on the particular "problems which minority group nurses have" within the profession.[37] The ANA, as the primary representative of the nursing profession, tied health to many of the tenets of the civil rights movement. The nursing profession advanced civil rights as a responsibility of the profession because many nurses viewed nursing as possessing a special and even privileged position within the social hierarchy of American society.[38]

In a 1956 editorial in the *American Journal of Nursing*, Grace Marr of the ANA argued that the duty of the "professions" in American society was to provide leadership and guidance in the effort to better society as a whole. Because of the status, leadership, and even social prestige attributed to professionals, members of the professions had an "obligation to provide leadership in the integration of all members . . . of society."[39] Their experience with "human relations," as Marr put it, placed members of the profession in a position wherein members of society emulated their behavior. Certainly, Marr's observations to that effect were not wrong. This was true within the African American community, where, for example, respected leaders who directed the course of community and civil rights activities were often doctors, lawyers, teachers, nurses, clergyman, and other professionals.[40]

The black nurse received greater respect than most other professionals because she "belonged to the community," working within it and on its behalf.[41] Black nurses were concerned not only with the health of the individual but also with how the individual's health affected the entire community. Marr's assertion that "a profession concerned with fulfilling its moral obligations [could not] afford to close its eyes to discriminatory practices within it or affecting it" implicitly linked civil rights to the caregiving mission of nurses. This was a recurring conversation in the pages of the *American Journal of Nursing* throughout the latter half of the 1950s.[42]

Within this agenda—the ANA's dedication to equality among its nurses and to guaranteeing equitable access to healthcare without regard to race, creed, color, or sex—becomes even more important to understanding how a gendered occupation was embroiled in the social transformations of the 1950s and 1960s. While guaranteeing equality or the end of discriminatory practices was nearly impossible on the community level, that the agenda of the ANA's leadership included this objective reveals the unbreakable link between the professional organization and social and political issues. This was best exemplified by the participation of nurses in the 1963 March on Washington. In an article titled "Nurses March and Care for Marchers," nurses were celebrated for both their dedication to equality and their ability to provide care during the event.[43]

Additionally, by formulating their activities in terms of healthcare needs, the American Nurses' Association and individual nurses pushed social boundaries to improve their professional and economic security. Historian Susan Rimby Leighow discusses this phenomenon in her essay on married women's labor-force participation. She argues that despite societal pressure to stay home in the 1950s, married female nurses used nursing shortages to justify their return to the workforce and, in doing so, forced hospitals to go out of their way to recruit and accommodate them.[44] This did not immediately change public opinion on married women's role in the labor force, but it was proof that a woman could function as both a mother and professional. Additionally, it eased the tension faced by those married women who either had to work or wanted to work. Finally, it provided one space wherein married women could not only win accommodations but could also challenge assumptions about who could offer care and at what stages in their lives they could offer it.

Reflections of these tensions in civil society were also evident in military nursing. Military preparedness and nursing shortages had demanded a revision of traditional conceptions of gender roles and racial hierarchies within the ranks of the ANC throughout the previous half-century. By the mid-1950s, nursing shortages accounted for three major changes to the 1901 formation of the Army Nurse Corps: the integration of the ANC and acceptance of African American female nurses during World War II, when racial policies restricted the inclusion of black female nurses prior to the 1940s; permanent integration of the nurse corps into the regular army, which provided job security and status to members of the nurse corps during World War II and in the postwar period; and the addition of male nurses into the Reserve Officers Corps in 1955, ending the exclusion of men from the nurse corps. Nevertheless, the ANC continued to struggle with race discrimination and gender inequality inside the organization and in response to events outside of it.

Challenges to Integration in the Army Nurse Corps

Integration problems within the ANC thwarted the military's attempt to stay out of civilian politics in all of its manifestations. On the surface, race integration appeared a success in the years since 1948, but as the experiences of nurses serving during the Korean conflict demonstrated, the reality proved inconsistent with military policy.[45] Race problems in local communities and among individual service members remained firmly attached to personal beliefs and cultural understandings. Even Walter Reed Army Hospital, the U.S. Army's medical institution near the nation's capital, was not immune to these conditions.

The 1955 experience of future Brig. Gen. Hazel Johnson-Brown provides a stunning example of the inconsistency between lived experience and military policy. When Johnson-Brown joined the ANC after several years in civilian nursing, integration had been a firmly established mandate for more than six years.[46] As an African American woman and professional nurse, Johnson-Brown could not have chosen a better time to join the armed forces. The nurse corps offered long-term career opportunities to women and minorities that had not existed even a decade before. Johnson-Brown's first assignment was at Walter Reed Army Hospital in Washington, D.C., in early 1955. The housemother in charge of the nursing quarters maintained racial segregation by assigning all the black nurses to one corner of one floor of the nursing residence. She assigned white nurses to the remaining parts of the building. While a white nurse and friend of Johnson-Brown's suggested they lodge a complaint because the two wished to room next to each other, Johnson-Brown told her friend to drop the complaint. She realized they could do very little without causing more problems for themselves and those around them. Johnson-Brown cautioned her friend about the need to "rise above" the behavior of the housemother.[47]

Coming on the heels of a national civil rights victory, the Walter Reed incident reminds us that policies or mandates did not guarantee an end to segregation or discrimination, nor were they something that whites accepted simply because the president, Congress, or the Supreme Court endorsed them. Johnson-Brown's response to the situation is interesting, in that it reveals some of the negotiations made by African Americans living through this period of transition in race relations. These negotiations were necessary in order to succeed in the military and civilian society.[48] Johnson-Brown understood that diehard supporters of segregation existed no matter where one was, and she even acknowledged that the incident at Walter Reed was "the behavior of [personnel] who had been there for years." When the housemother retired, the practice of segregating the nurses by race stopped. This whole business of race, Johnson-Brown suggested, "stems from the fact there is a belief [that] because there is color to your skin, you are lesser in quality. Something less about you."[49] Even while African Americans took to the streets in greater force to demand equality and became less willing to accept injustice, negotiations like Brown's were the only way most African American men and women could protect themselves.[50]

Like Johnson-Brown's suggestion to "rise above," ongoing racial tensions revealed that African American service members also understood that a different standard of behavior existed for them. In order to succeed and navigate the milieu of race discrimination they needed to monitor themselves and the behaviors of their fellow service members. During her first tour of duty overseas in 1963, Clara Adams-Ender remembers having to report to the tent of an African American nurse captain. This captain imparted what Adams-Ender believed was the most important advice and orders she received during her early career.

> You will not, Lieutenant, do anything in this place to embarrass or discredit your fellow Negro Officers. . . . We've spent a lot of time and effort making sure that we have a good reputation over here and we intend to keep things that way. You may see other officers saying and doing all kinds of things, but remember that I am personally going to be watching you. . . . Negro officers are watched more closely than white officers. That's just the way it is.[51]

The "unvarnished fact of life" that Adams-Ender remembered as holding true throughout her military career beginning in the early 1960s reveals the harsh reality of integration. Integration as a path to equality or an end to race discrimination was difficult to achieve even as Adams-Ender's story reveals a successful military career. The experiences of African American female nurses serving in the ANC provide one way to scrutinize the complicated negotiations made by racial minorities and men and women in the post–World War II era of social justice.

The history of the ANC in this period also highlights tensions and conflicts beyond *racial* integration in the postwar era. The integration of men into the ANC proved a fraught undertaking and one that held significance for broader struggles for gender equality. The 1955 amendment to the Army-Navy Nurse Act of 1947 brought men into the ranks of the ANC. While heralded as a milestone in the progress of American nursing, it did little to formalize or guarantee equality between the sexes. A closer examination of the amendment and its implementation reveals both an acceptance of a traditional sexual division of labor and the difficulties in attempting to balance this with the mission of the nurse corps. It would be simple to view the acceptance of male nurses as an example of the military's or society's approval of redefined gender roles, but such a conclusion would fail to recognize the historic circumstances that underlay this approval. It would also be easy—yet incorrect—to assume that the Army Nurse Corps' eventual support of the 1955 legislation meant that the organization was a socially progressive branch of military. The ANC was not a liberal organization attempting to challenge gender norms. The acceptance of both men and women into the ANC did eventually lead to advances in equitable gender relations, but this needs to be understood, at least in part, in the context of military need. The army saw the addition of men as a practical matter, shoring up their numbers and broadening where and when they could provide care for soldiers and their families.

The addition of male nurses to the ANC did not immediately accomplish the full and equal integration of male nurses. Instead, the amendment was in many ways a partial integration of men into the female-controlled organization. As the previous chapter revealed, male nurses accepted as officers in the ANC became commissioned officers of the reserve corps, not the regular army.[52] The Military Occupational Specialties (MOS) designation of (MN) for Male Nurse further differentiated male nurses from female nurses for the first couple of years of male enlistment in the ANC.[53] While not the advantageous outcome that many hoped for, it was the only compromise available to get men into the nurse corps. Congresswoman Frances Payne Bolton reminded LeRoy Craig and others of this fact when she wrote in 1958: "It was not until we suggested exactly that, that the Army would consider the matter at all."[54] Indeed, years of war and associated nursing shortages could not overcome the tenacity of either the conventional view of nurses as women or the fierce determination of some female nurses to protect what they viewed as women's domain. Securing commission in the reserve corps for men was the result of nearly four decades of work, and yet, both men and women held ambivalent views of this accomplishment.

Distinct differences between male and female nurses who chose to join the ANC also accounted for tension between the two groups. Female nurses first entering the ranks of the ANC were young and single, often in their early twenties, and joining the military directly or within a few years of completing their nursing programs. In contrast, many of the male nurses who joined the nurse corps were often a little older, in their mid-to-late twenties, and had either previous experience in the military or in a civilian medical field.[55] In addition, although "the usual stereotypes of men being homosexuals . . . who went into nursing" persisted, a large number of these men were married or soon married after joining the ANC. Marriage to a woman—an outward appearance of heterosexuality—countered the argument that male nurses were homosexuals.[56] Further highlighting the differences between these male and female nurses were the types of jobs that attracted male nurses. Surgery, psychiatry, and anesthesia all attracted men in high numbers and emphasized how even within an occupation historically gendered as female, the types of nursing activities could become gendered as well. Anesthesia in particular drew a large majority of men. As one male nurse explained, "It is high tech in a lot of ways. So that's kind of appealing and that's one of the reasons I think that there are more men in it than in any other specialties except psychiatry."[57] The scientific or technical side of nursing also drew men because of its closeness to the work of physicians. "You know, it's really nice because you get to take care of people, and you don't have to go [to school] as long as a physician, and you don't have total responsibility like physicians," remembers one male nurse who was advised by a friend to consider anesthesia.[58]

Commissions in the reserve corps, however, meant that male nurses remained a minority in the corps, with little possibility of dominating or leading the group in the future. The reserve corps also created an opportunity for the ANC to exploit male nurses. For example, between 1955 and 1959, nearly three hundred men applied for appointment in the reserve corps, and nearly three-fourths of those men were accepted and serving on concurrent active duty.[59] This meant that while most reserve nurses served on active duty only during emergencies or in times of severe shortages, most male nurses served on active duty almost from the beginning of their enlistment. Concurrent active duty not only defeated the main purpose of the reserve corps, but the situation was, according to one nurse, a "disadvantage to the . . . individual male nurse."[60] Whereas the army viewed male nurses who entered active duty as "long-term career" members of the service, their status as reservists and the fact that many of the male nurses were older meant that even in promotions, men lagged behind women.[61]

Duty assignments further highlighted the continuing divide between female and male army nurses. Although one army report on the use of male nurses in the ANC suggested that "the field of nursing in the public mind is no longer considered solely a women's profession," the assignment of male nurse officers revealed that this perception persisted. For example, in smaller hospitals that treated both male and female patients and where nurses covered several wards, the sole use of male nurses was regarded as impossible. Social custom, the report noted, required that female nurses be present in the care of women.[62] Nevertheless, by the late 1950s this was changing in the civilian nursing profession, as "it became mandatory to do OB/GYN because it became part of the nursing boards in order to become an RN."[63] That the military declined to support caregiving by male nurses, regardless of the patient's sex, further illustrated the military's struggle with ongoing social understanding of the need to "protect" [female] patients against any behavior that would be deemed as inappropriate. It is noteworthy—or perhaps understandable, given the image of women in American society—that the military mentions no similar dilemma of protection for female doctors.[64] Nowhere in the debate about commissioning female doctors does anyone suggest that there might be a problem with women doctors providing patient care because of their sex. It was, in short, inconceivable that protection through the assistance of male nurses would be necessary for female doctors. Women doctors, as caregivers, did not need protection when working with the bodies of male patients any more than female nurses did. This question emerged only in relation to male nurses. Thus, we can infer that limited duty assignments for men benefited women nurses by rendering them nearly indispensable.

Special duty assignments for male nurses provided men some opportunities not open to female nurses, however. Male nurses allowed the army to broaden its use of medical personnel in areas deemed too dangerous for female nurses. This fulfilled a decade's long push to protect female nurses from duty that placed them in any sort of peril.[65] Mildred I. Clark, ANC chief in the mid-1960s, remembers explaining the support male nurses could provide: "Suppose you had a combat situation and couldn't assign women without weapons to take care of things, and you had to furnish somebody from your unit to go and take the security aspects of this hospital. What would you do? Would you rather have male nurses who could do this or furnish your own men? They said, we never thought about that. That's fine, we agree with you."[66] Female nurses did not undergo weapons training in the army until 1964. The expectation was that men nurses would provide a dual role for the military as both nurse and soldier. The acceptance of this dual role was a dramatic change for an army that had believed strongly in the separation of nurse and soldier during World War II.[67] The assignment of male nurses to army airborne duty revealed just how far the military had come in its thinking on the usefulness of male nurses. It reinforced the notion that male nurses were not only necessary to the ANC but also helped carve out a niche for male nurses that was fully in line with conventional gender roles. In 1956 three male nurses reported for airborne training at Fort Campbell, Kentucky.[68] Two years later, the army officially assigned three male nurses to each of the two medical units attached to the airborne divisions.[69] Beyond their training as ANC officers, these men had to train to become part of this division, which included jumping out of airplanes. This, as well as the combat nature of the airborne division, originally kept the army from assigning any female nurses to the airborne medical units.[70] The addition of male nurses provided valuable healthcare to the men in airborne, but also strengthened the argument for the full integration of male nurses into the ANC.

Protectionist arguments were used to strengthen the position of male nurses in the ANC throughout the late 1950s. Realistically, the ability of the army to execute a solution to concerns about female nurses in combat-forward hospitals was difficult to achieve. Nevertheless, conservative thinking continued to clash with caregiving and gender roles in the practical administration of the ANC. Col. Margaret Harper, ANC chief from 1959 to 1963, stated that duty in forward areas often required "officers highly qualified in a clinical specialty." This included nurses trained to work in the operating room and in anesthesia. Although a large number of men went into specialties such as anesthesia, there were not enough male nurses to meet this demand, but there were plenty of female nurses to supply these services. It would be impossible for the ANC to support the assigning of only male nurses in combat areas. Further, Harper noted that many commanders in forward areas continued to comment on the "high morale when female Army Nurse Corps officers were with these units." Many of these commanders believed that the will and strength to continue to fight was something that only a woman, because of the unique qualifications of her sex, could provide to fighting men. Whether there was scientific proof to back this did not matter as much as the fact that thinking in these terms remained strong. This was encouraged not only by men but also by women in defending the unique role of women in nursing. Harper's comments reveal the difficulty in reconciling the realities of combat needs with public or military dogma concerning female nurses in combat zones. The acceptance of male nurses more widely in civilian and military nursing, however, supported a slow transformation of these reservations in the late 1950s. Thus, despite her comments on women's special ability to enhance military morale, Colonel Harper also acknowledged, in her final comments on male nurses, that sex alone should not determine assignment in the ANC. Instead, experience, training, and education should frame the basis for any assignments.[71]

Harper's emphasis on qualifications rather than sex in the assignment of duty presents a unique opportunity to examine how the ANC thought about equity among its members. One of the largest obstacles to the acceptance of male nurses, especially during the early 1950s campaign to amend the Army-Navy Nurse Act of 1947, stemmed from the chief nurses' concerns about benefits. Although some women nurse officers understood and even accepted as fair that male nurses received benefits they themselves did not have access to, others pointed to the dangerous and discriminatory environment this would create. Therefore, many of the senior officers supported the acceptance of men into the ANC only if equitable benefits were available to both men and women.[72] This view was certainly contrary to widely held and accepted practices of differential compensation between men and women in both the military and civilian society, but given both the overwhelming majority of women in the profession and the commonly acknowledged reality that nursing was regarded as a female occupation, chief officers expected access to the same benefits nonetheless. If "qualifications" should be the basis for unbiased assignments, as Harper suggested in her 1959 report, the military's refusal to change its policies with respect to benefits proved contradictory to this thinking. It demonstrated, instead, a male-biased adherence to conventional economic and labor practices that benefited men even while the army championed nursing as an opportunity for women's economic independence and advancement.[73]

Concerns raised by female nurse chiefs in 1950 regarding the acceptance of male nurses proved an unfortunate reality with the addition of male nurses to the organization in 1955.[74] Although they were members of the Reserve Officers Corps, many of whom served on active duty as well, male nurse officers received benefits that were not available to the highest-ranking female members of the ANC. Married male nurse officers received family quarters or the equivalent allowance to live elsewhere and were allowed dependents under age eighteen. In contrast, the ANC denied admission to any married woman who wished to join in the 1950s. Those who were already nurse corps officers had to seek permission to marry.[75] Further, under normal circumstances married female nurse officers did not receive family quarters. They received only a housing allowance if their husbands were completely dependent on them. Spousal dependency was something they needed to prove before they could qualify for the same benefits men received without difficulty. To add to the already imbalanced dealings between the two sexes, female nurses also could not have dependents under the age of eighteen during the late 1950s and early 1960s. These discrepancies reveal the army's reluctance to acknowledge changes that had taken place within the civilian nursing profession. The army remained firmly attached to its view on gender relations, as evidenced by its refusal to integrate male nurses into the regular army while continuing to use them on active duty, and by their refusal to grant female nurse officers the same benefits as male officers. Attempts on the part of nurses and nurse supporters to redefine these circumstances emerged as the country entered a period of unprecedented social change.

Male and female nurses were firmly engaged in a discussion about fair and equal treatment and discrimination in employment long before the passage of the Civil Rights Act in 1964. Gender roles and equality continued to be a major topic in discussions about nurse recruitment and integration in the ANC as second-wave feminists' ideas challenged the gender status quo. Within the context of critical nursing shortages—thousands of World War II–era nurses retired in the late 1950s and early 1960s—these discussions were important in understanding the nurse corps actions with regard to nursing employment. Army nurse leaders faced a deficit of nearly two thousand nurses in 1963. Recruitment measures in the form of educational support and financial and other career incentives, however, focused largely on the recruitment of young, white, female nurses, according to historian Kara Dixon Vuic. Recruitment materials throughout the 1960s failed to incorporate minority female or male nurses, with few exceptions.[76] This suggests that, in general, even with the integration of African American female nurses and the acceptance of male nurses, an underlying image about who was a nurse remained.[77]

This traditional image of nurses and persistent gender conventions presented a challenge to the equality of female nurses within the military and the ANC. Long-established policies about marriage, dependents, and benefits remained even after Title VII deemed sex discrimination illegal in employment. At a military medical conference in 1964, ANC chief Mildred I. Clark expressed hope that the surgeon general would soon overturn the policy against married women applying to the regular army, for example.[78] In December 1964, the military finally acknowledged married women as an untapped labor pool for the ANC and revised its policy to allow married women to apply for appointment in the regular army. In that same year, the military also reduced the minimum age of dependents allowed for women from eighteen to fifteen. However, this rule continued to apply only to female nurses, not male nurses, for example.[79] This revealed a persistent bias in some quarters that only women of certain ages or circumstances should work outside of the home—women with no children or older children and women who were older or unmarried.

Five years after male nurses became members of the Reserve Officers Corps of the ANC the number of men on active duty remained high. Surgeon General Leonard Heaton noted that as of May 1961, 251 male nurses served as reserve officers. This was about 5 percent of the total male nurse population in the United States.[80] Heaton suggested that, given the valuable service male nurses provided to the nurse corps, the time had come for the Department of the Army either to propose or support legislation for the addition of male nurses to the regular army. This was the first full support from a surgeon general that male nurses received for their campaign. Heaton cautiously suggested that while no set quota of male nurses should be written into the legislation, a limit to the number of male nurses accepted into the nurse corps should be "administratively imposed by the Secretary of the Army as required and appropriate." Undoubtedly, this language does suggest a quota on the number of male nurses allowed into the regular army and restricted the opportunity of men wanting to enter the ANC. In the words of the surgeon general, this method of employing male nurses in the regular army also kept "the Corps a predominately female organization."[81]

Given the difficulty with recruiting and the continued restrictions placed on the female nurse population, the opinions of the surgeon general seemed contradictory. Mildred I. Clark even expressed the hope that male nurse commissions in the regular army would alleviate the strain of the nursing shortage and explained to members of the medical staff the desire for congressional legislation.[82] Congresswoman Frances Bolton took up the call and again introduced legislation to commission male nurses into the regular army in 1961 and again in 1963. However, as with her previous experiences with male nurse legislation, the bills failed to pass.[83] Male nurse integration looked less likely than it had in years. Even after the passage of the Civil Rights Act, male nurses confronted the disadvantages of gender conventions and their effect on the nursing profession. As had been the case since World War II, however, war helped shape and refine the debate about equality, especially gender equality, in the ANC.

Lyndon Johnson's 1965 call for troops in Vietnam found the ANC once again in immediate need of active-duty nurses. Although the army had nurses stationed in Vietnam since 1956 and more than two hundred by 1965, Johnson's call for a troop increase meant that the few hundred nurses serving in Vietnam could not meet all the in-country nursing needs. In fact, by the summer of 1965 the ANC had to employ nearly two thousand civilian nurses to meet its demands domestically and abroad. To guarantee adequate nursing support, Johnson issued a special draft for male nurses in April 1966. The Department of Defense requested seven hundred male nurses for the army and another two hundred for the navy.[84] Reminiscent of the draft proposal for female nurses during World War II, Johnson's Special Call 38 did not face the same public backlash as the 1945 draft proposal. This was because men were subject to the draft, and the draft of male nurses did not have the same gendered connotations as the prospect of drafting women into the military. However, even with a draft, the military did not ease the nursing shortage.[85]

Congress had already begun seriously debating the commissioning of male nurses in the regular army by the time Johnson called a draft for male nurses. Reports before the House and Senate revealed that since 1955 the military had closely studied the effectiveness of male nurses. The results found that "male nurses . . . proved that they can make valuable contributions to the missions of the military services." Furthermore, the report noted that commissioning male nurses as regular officers was beneficial for the army: "Male nurses, in many instances, are able to remain in service longer than women nurses. Marriage and the coming of family, for example, do not terminate a male nurse's career, as it does with female nurses in the Armed Forces."[86] While certainly not imagining an ANC without female nurses, male nurses made up about one-fifth of the entire nurse corps strength by 1966. The congressional reports are interesting because they suggest that the addition of male nurses was attractive for the very reasons that kept men from the nurse corps in earlier periods: their sex, and a belief in distinctive gender behaviors and roles. The ANC and the U.S. military's own policies, until 1964, hindered some women from having long-term careers in the service; these policies suggested that a woman had to forgo children and possibly marriage in order to have long-term career prospects. Nevertheless, Congress and the military had finally recognized that the race or sex of the nurse could no longer undermine their need for nurses. After several failed attempts to legislate the integration of male nurses in the ANC, nursing activists cheered the passage of Public Law 89-609 in July 1966.[87] This law provided male nurses with commissions into the regular army, but, more important, it indicated a fundamental shift in the way the U.S. Army conceptualized nursing in the military.

Conclusion

The War Department [the Army] has maintained
throughout the emergency and present
war that it is not the appropriate medium
for affecting social readjustments.

—Robert F. Patterson to Governor Chauncey Sparks,
September 1, 1944

Forty years after asking the Red Cross and the army to change their policies on the acceptance of male nurses, men had achieved full military standing and recognition in the ANC. Along with changes to the acceptance of female nurses beginning in 1964—the acceptance of married women, for example—the ANC could, in 1966, claim to be a race- and sex-inclusive organization. Yet many of these changes were pragmatic rather than politically motivated on the part of the ANC. This story reveals an organization bound reluctantly yet intimately to social-justice activism, shaped by war and military preparedness and hindered by nursing shortages. The history of the ANC suggests another way of understanding the civil rights movement of the twentieth century, one that views the movement as several overlapping movements that were at times progressive and conservative, whose actors were concerned with not only race discrimination but gender inequality, sex discrimination, and economic and labor equity.

While promoting itself as a conservative institution, the ANC became an organization that challenged traditional values and cultural understandings of race and gender differences that shaped the social hierarchy in American society. The very mission of the ANC, to provide care to soldiers and military service to the nation, mirrored values materially and symbolically important in American society. However, even before its formal establishment, the challenge of fulfilling those values within the confines of acceptable social roles and practices placed the ANC in an unusual position. From the end of the nineteenth century through the second half of the twentieth, the organization played a part in confronting the presumptive roles of women and men, conservative beliefs about race, and service to the country.

Nursing allowed women to carve out a legitimate niche for themselves in the military. Within the framework of a gendered occupation, they used the military to mount a slow but consistent fight for autonomy and professional recognition that translated to a more concerted effort for women's equality. The same can be said about racial civil rights. African American female nurses saw in the ANC's mission another opportunity to push for integration and equality as the nation fought to defend the principles of democracy throughout the world. Additionally, the attempt by male nurses to breach this all-female bastion allowed male and female nurses the chance to negotiate a new level of gender equity in the 1950s and 1960s. From 1939 to 1969, changes to ANC policies unmasked a larger reality on the issue of equality and rights in American society. The civilian nursing profession mirrored attempts to redefine race and gender roles during and after wartime. As a whole, the nursing profession exposes a movement for social justice that was simultaneously progressive, conservative, and continuously evolving.

In the years immediately following the passage of Public Law 89-609, the ANC struggled to maintain advances in race and gender equality. In the context of a transitioning civil rights movement that followed the passage of the 1964 Civil Rights Act, gender conventions still shaped the experiences of male and female nurses. In 1968, for example, at the height of the Vietnam War, the army deployed several "all male" nursing units for the purpose of increased mobility in combat zones. These all-male units presented some problems for the ANC, and the chief nurse found it necessary to reassign several of the male nurses. When questioned about the reassignment, one commander stated: "We need the females for 'bargaining power' to obtain additional support. These men were wonderful in the beginning, but even the Chief Nurse stated that they needed females to maintain adequate standards."[1] As it had since World War II and the Korean War, the allusion to the inferiority of male nurse training and education, as well as the "need" for women to care for male soldiers, remained strong even after the integration of male nurses into the regular army. The chief of the ANC later insisted, "You will [not] find any prejudice against male nurses in the Army . . . [yet] we do have prejudice against 'poor nursing care' rendered by either sex." However, the suggestion that the female nurse was necessary to maintain standards and to be used as a "bargaining tool" reveals an understanding that, without women, nursing and the ability to provide care falls apart. Further complicating the position of male nurses was the continued prejudice and suspicion against them. In 1972 the Office of the Surgeon General received a phone call from a commanding officer whose unit served primarily dependents of military personnel. During this conversation, Colonel Capel requested that no male nurses be assigned to his unit because many of the nearly three thousand dependents they served objected to male nurse care.[2] Colonel Capel's request may be location specific, but it reveals the ongoing unease that male nurses elicited in some individuals. Under these and similar circumstances it was difficult for the ANC to assure the fair distribution of duty assignment between men and women in the military.

Female nurses also struggled with gender inequities. Despite their overwhelming majority in the ANC, female nurses still faced gender-based restrictions that were more readily apparent in light of male nurse integration in the regular army. Although the ANC changed its policy to allow for the acceptance of married nurses into the organization in 1964, it was seven more years before the nurse corps removed all dependent restrictions for female nurses. Seven years is not so significant when examined within the context of the women's rights movement of the 1960s and 1970s, but given that such a decision affected the opportunities of the majority of nurses who populated the ANC, this was a considerable amount of time. Until the early 1970s only women whose dependents were older than age fifteen or who had no dependents could apply to the ANC. Male nurses, in contrast, had no restrictions on dependents. Furthermore, it was not until 1967 that restrictions on the promotion of female officers in the ANC changed in any significant manner. The removal of promotion restrictions meant that women were finally evaluated using the same guidelines for promotion as men in the regular army.[3] This policy should have been in place once the ANC became a permanent part of the regular army in 1947.

Integration also failed to resolve the recruitment problems and nursing shortages that remained a constant for the ANC. The opening of the nurse corps to men as well as to a greater number of women in the 1960s did not completely alleviate either problem. To make matters worse, after years of relatively successful integration and recruitment of minority nurses, the ANC found itself charged with discrimination against African Americans. In 1972 a group calling itself U-BAD (United Blacks Against Discrimination) argued that nurse corps shortages stemmed from racist recruitment policies at the Walter Reed Army Institute of Nursing (WRAIN).[4] The protestors staged a brief but radical campaign aimed at threatening WRAIN into accepting more black students into the nursing program. The ANC responded to these charges by forming a minority recruitment committee and was able to increase the recruitment of minority nurses in the years following the protest.[5]

The successes and struggles of the ANC from the 1950s to the 1970s also shed light on critical moments in the history of the nursing profession. These decades witnessed the professionalization of nursing, with education and nursing standards firmly attached to university-level advanced-degree programs, even while nurses themselves continued to debate the term "professional."[6] Magnified within the civilian nursing profession were the same struggles over employment opportunities, advancements in nursing care, and changes to nursing education requirements that the Army Nurse Corps debated as they strove for full professionalization. Nevertheless, even the American Nurses' Association, which promoted itself as the national nursing advocacy group, struggled in its duty to support all nurses. Although dedicated to the equality of opportunity for all nurses, charges of discrimination in the profession and organization were a recurring subject, as they had been for the ANC. By the 1970s male nurses and African Americans nurses alike established their own professional organizations. These are the National Black Nurses Association (1971) and the American Assembly for Men in Nursing (1974), respectively.[7] The establishment of a new black nursing association is especially telling, as it was the dissolution of the National Association of Colored Graduate Nurses in 1950 that heralded a new era of racial cooperation in the profession.

In the twenty-first century, the consequences of the ANC nurse integration campaigns present a complex image of the fight for equality and social justice. They reveal the unfinished and, at times, the tenuous nature of the fight for race and gender equality in the late twentieth century. The integration campaigns pursued by female and male nurses expose a civil rights movement beyond the question of race. Certainly, race equality and racial justice dominated the movement throughout the mid-twentieth century; however, as the history of the ANC demonstrates, redefining gender roles and a push for labor and economic equality also played a role in broadening the terms of social justice. The appointment of the first male chief of the ANC in 2000 signaled an astonishing progressive move on the part of the ANC, but what is perhaps even more impressive is the fact that by 2003, male nurses made up 34 percent of the corps, and African American women 18 percent.[8] Despite its desire otherwise, the Army Nurse Corps' and U.S. military's attempt to preserve a conservative persona throughout the mid- to late twentieth century was consistently challenged by nursing shortages, war, and a push for social justice in civil society. In their attempt to remain separated from the "social readjustments" taking place in civilian society, the ANC and the U.S. Army often found themselves at the very center of the conversation, if not shaping the conversation.

Facts about Negro Nurses and the War

Prepared jointly by the National Association of Colored Graduate Nurses and the National Nursing Council for War Service, 1790 Broadway, New York, N.Y.

		Number	Percentage
(1a) Active graduate nurses estimated as of January 1, 1945		274,405	100.0
(1b) Active Negro graduate nurses included in (a)	(est.)	8,000	2.9
(2a) Nurses now in army		44,000	100.0
(2b) Negro nurses now in army included in (2a)	(est.)	330	0.75
(3a) Nurses now in navy		9,165	100.0
(3b) Negro nurses now in navy		—	0.0
(4a) All active graduate nurses		274,405	100.0
(4b) Nurses now in army and navy (2a and 3a)		53,165	19.0
(4c) Nurses needed in addition by army and navy		18,335	6.5
(5a) Active Negro graduate nurses	(est.)	8,000	100.0
(5b) Negro nurses in army		333	4.1
(6a) Total number of men in army	(more than)	8,000,000	100.0
(6b) Total number of Negro men in army		701,678	8.7

Some Conclusions Drawn from the Figures Above

There are only one-tenth as many Negro nurses in the Army Nurse Corps, in proportion to the total corps, as there are Negroes in the army as a whole.

Basis:	87 out of 1,000 in the army are Negroes (6b)
But only:	8 out of 1,000 in the Army Nurse Corps are Negroes (2b)

In proportion to their numbers, Negro nurses are supplying less than one-quarter as many numbers to the Army and Navy Nurse Corps as in the nursing profession as a whole.

Basis:	190 out of every 1,000 nurses are in the army and navy (4b)
But only:	41 out of every 1,000 Negro nurses are in the army and navy (5b)

If as many Negro nurses—in proportion to their numbers—as white nurses were accepted by the army and navy, there would be 1,520 Negro nurses in the army and navy instead of the 330 in the army.

Basis:	19 percent of all active nurses are in the army or navy (4b)
	19 percent of all active Negro nurses would be 1,520 (1b)

Note: The statements above are not to be interpreted as an argument for the quota system but instead as a measure of a failure to fully utilize Negro nurse resources.

Male Nurse Population, 1943

Table B.1   The U.S. Census number of men nurses (graduates and students) in the United States.

Year	Number
1940	8,072
1930	5,452
1920	5,464
1910	5,819

1930 Census, vol. 5, p. 20; and 1940 Census, series P-11, summary pp. 3, 5. Reprinted from *Facts about Nursing*, 1950, p. 12.

Table B.2   Registered Men Nurses in the Armed Forces—January 1943 (based on questionnaires returned by 1,269 registered men nurses). Number in the Armed Forces.

Service	Number	Percent
All Services	320	100.0
Army	172	53.8
Navy	136	42.5
Coast Guard	10	3.1
Marine Corps	2	0.6

"Men Nurses and the Armed Services," *American Journal of Nursing* v. 43, no. 12 (December 1943), p. 1067. Reprinted from *Facts about Nursing*, 1950, p. 12. Courtesy of Wolters Kluwer Heath, Inc.

Table B.3   Age range of men in armed forces

Age Range	Number	Percent
Total Reporting	320	100.0
Under 25 years	93	29.1
25–29 years	126	39.4
30–34 years	63	19.7
35–39 years	28	8.7
40 and over	10	3.1

Reprinted from *Facts about Nursing*, 1950, p. 12. Courtesy of the American Nurses' Association.

APPENDIX C

African American Nurse Population, 1940

Negro Nurses (Graduate and Student)—1940

State	Total	Women	Men
Alabama	415	400	15
Arizona	7	6	1
Arkansas	62	62	0
California	155	153	2
Colorado	1	1	0
Connecticut	7	7	0
Delaware	9	9	0
District of Columbia	288	286	2
Florida	282	270	12
Georgia	577	569	8
Idaho	0	0	0
Illinois	268	263	5
Indiana	40	39	1
Iowa	1	1	0
Kansas	37	37	0
Kentucky	94	91	3
Louisiana	127	126	1
Maine	1	1	0
Maryland	130	126	4
Massachusetts	55	53	2
Michigan	120	117	3
Minnesota	5	5	0
Mississippi	131	128	3
Missouri	431	431	0
Montana	0	0	0
Nebraska	1	1	0
Nevada	0	0	0

State	Total	Women	Men
New Hampshire	0	0	0
New Jersey	110	106	4
New Mexico	0	0	0
New York	1,723	1,714	9
North Carolina	481	474	7
North Dakota	0	0	0
Ohio	118	115	3
Oklahoma	55	54	1
Oregon	1	0	1
Pennsylvania	205	200	5
Rhode Island	3	3	0
South Carolina	259	255	4
South Dakota	0	0	0
Tennessee	266	262	4
Texas	259	247	12
Utah	0	0	0
Vermont	1	1	0
Virginia	414	407	7
Washington	2	2	0
West Virginia	46	45	1
Wisconsin	5	3	2
Wyoming	0	0	0
Total—United States	7,192	7,065	127

Source: U.S. Census, 1940. "Third Series Population Bulletin." Reprinted from *Facts about Nursing,* 1940.

Male and African American
Nurse Population, 1950

Table D.5   Men Student Nurses Admitted and Graduated During the Year, 1945–1950, and Number Enrolled on January 1.

Year	Admitted	Graduated	Enrolled on January 1
1950	. . .	. . .	900
1949	398	136	719
1948	470	28	455
1947	334	42	. . .
1946	. . .	36	72
1945	42	28	. . .

Source: NLNE, 1950. Reprinted from *Facts about Nursing*, 1950, p. 38. Courtesy of the National League for Nursing.

Table D.6   Negro Student Nurses Admitted and Graduated During the Year, 1945–1950, and Number Enrolled on January 1.

Year	Admitted	Graduate	Enrolled on January 1
1950	. . .	. . .	3,076
1949	1,383	507	2,504
1948	1,262	597	2,255
1947	1,001	592	. . .
1946	. . .	540	2,281
1945	821	520	. . .

Source: NLNE, 1950. Reprinted from *Facts about Nursing*, 1950, p. 38. Courtesy of the National League for Nursing.

Notes

Introduction

1. Brig. Gen. Bettye H. Simmons, "Message from the Chief, Army Nurse Corps," The Connection, Retired Army Nurse Corps Association 25, no.1 (March 2000): 2, as quoted in Dorothy B. Pocklington, ed., *Heritage of Leadership: Army Nurse Corps Biographies* (Ellicott City, Md.: Aldot, 2004), 125.

2. According to the Army Nurse Corps records, by 2003 male nurses composed 34 percent of the Corps, African American women 18 percent. See Army Nurse Corps Newsletter Historical Articles: "Proud to Serve: African American Army Nurse Corps Officers" and "Proud to Serve: The Evolution of Male Army Nurse Corps Officers," available at http://history.amedd.army.mil/ANCWebsite/articles/blackhistory.html and http://history.amedd.army.mil/ANCWebsite/articles/malenurses.html, respectively (accessed August 12, 2014).

3. Susan Hirsch, *After the Strike: A Century of Labor Struggle at Pullman* (Urbana: University of Illinois Press, 2003).

4. Linda Kerber, "Separate Spheres, Female Worlds, Woman's Place: The Rhetoric of Women's History," *Journal of American History* 75, no. 1 (June 1988): 10–17 and 38–39; Joan Wallach Scott, *Gender and the Politics of History* (New York: Columbia University Press, 1999).

5. R. W. Connell, *Masculinities* (Berkeley: University of California Press, 1995), 68.

6. Linda Kerber, *No Constitutional Right to Be Ladies: Women and the Obligations of Citizenship* (New York: Hill and Wang, 1999).

7. Here, I am applying the work of Mary Dudziak to examine the pervasive way that fears about communist subversion shaped or hindered the strategies available to individuals and groups who challenged the acceptable behaviors, life choices, and

rights in postwar America. Mary Dudziak, *Cold War Civil Rights: Race and the Image of American Democracy* (Princeton, N.J.: Princeton University Press, 2000).

8. Scott, *Gender*; Alice Kessler-Harris, *In Pursuit of Equity: Women, Men, and the Quest for Economic Citizenship in 20th-Century America* (New York: Oxford University Press, 2001); Joanne Meyerowitz, ed. *Not June Cleaver: Women and Gender in Postwar America, 1945–1960, Critical Perspectives on the Past* (Philadelphia: Temple University Press, 1994); Kerber, *No Constitutional Right.*

9. Susan M. Reverby, *Ordered to Care: The Dilemma of American Nursing, 1850–1945*, Cambridge Studies in the History of Medicine (Cambridge: Cambridge University Press, 1987); Darlene Clark Hine, *Black Women in White: Racial Conflict and Cooperation in the Nursing Profession, 1890–1950*, Blacks in the Diaspora (Bloomington: Indiana University Press, 1989); Susan Smith, *Sick and Tired of Being Sick and Tired: Black Women's Health in America, 1890–1950* (Philadelphia: University of Pennsylvania Press, 1995); Barbara Melosh, *"The Physician's Hand": Work Culture and Conflict in American Nursing* (Philadelphia: Temple University Press, 1982); Kimberly Jensen, *Mobilizing Minerva: American Women in the First World War* (Urbana: University of Illinois Press, 2008).

10. In 1930 members of a special committee of the American Nurses' Association presented a report requesting the replacement of "Sub-professional service" classification for nursing with "Professional." They argued that according to government classification in 1930, the work nursing did was professional and considered part of the professional class in forty-six states, so therefore the occupation should be listed as a "profession." American Nurses' Association, "Brief and Specifications for Civilian Nursing Service in the Federal Government," [1930] *American Nurses' Association*, Howard Gotlieb Research Center, Boston University, box 158, folder 3 [hereinafter HGARC].

11. In a historic overview of nurses who served during the Civil War, Stimson and Thompson noted remarks made during an 1890 discussion on passing legislation to form a nurse corps. They noted that the "discussion" focused solely on white females and remarked that leaving out men and women of color was "unjust discrimination against" the individuals who had served as nurses during the Civil War. This reveals an early discussion of the systematic barring of women of color and men in the nursing profession. Julia Stimson and Ethel C. Thompson, "Women Nurses with the Union Forces during the Civil War," *Military Surgeon* (February 1928): 221–22.

12. Minority nurses included not only African American female nurses and other nurses of color but also male nurses who were in the minority in the profession.

Chapter 1. The Politics of Intimate Care

1. Jane E. Schultz, "The Inhospitable Hospital: Gender and Professionalism in Civil War Medicine," *Signs* (Winter 1992): 366.

2. For information on antebellum gender behavior see, Jane E. Schultz, *Women at the Front: Hospital Workers in Civil War America* (Chapel Hill: University of North Carolina Press, 2004), xxi–ii.

3. Casey Wood, "The Nurse and the Medical Man," *American Journal of Nursing* 4, no. 4 (January 1904): 279–81; and "Organized Opposition to Nursing Progress," in "Editorial Comments," *American Journal of Nursing* 10, no. 1 (October 1909): 5.

4. According to Reverby, "by the early nineteenth century, nursing began to emerge in the more formal urban marketplace as a category in the expanding field of domestic service"; here, however, it had a poor reputation and was often viewed as an inferior and less-than-respectable "paid" occupation for women of a certain class and/or background. Reverby, *Ordered to Care*, 1–2 and 13–16; and Philip Kalisch and Beatrice Kalisch, *The Advance of American Nursing* (Philadelphia: Lippincott, 1995), 26–27.

5. Elizabeth D. Leonard, *Yankee Women: Gender Battles in the Civil War* (New York: Norton, 1994), introduction; and Schultz, *Women at the Front*, xxiii.

6. Paul H. Ringer, "The Responsibility of the Trained Nurse to the Community," *American Journal of Nursing* 10, no. 12 (September 1910): 934.

7. Nursing history is not just women's history or labor history; it is also gender history, race history, and class history. Melosh, *"The Physician's Hand,"* 6–9.

8. Kalisch and Kalisch, *Advance of American Nursing*, 30–32.

9. The diseases most likely to be contracted by soldiers in British hospitals included dysentery, typhoid, and cholera, all of which can be avoided simply with better sanitary measures. Ibid., 32.

10. Ibid., 36.

11. Ibid., 32.

12. In 1860, Nightingale opened the Nightingale Training School for Nurses at St. Thomas Hospital in London. Her belief in nursing as the exclusive domain of women—"God's work, in simplicity and singleness of heart"—gained traction among American women looking to promote nursing as a career option for women. Florence Nightingale, *Notes on Nursing: What It Is, and What It Is Not* (1859; repr. Philadelphia: Lippincott, 1992), 1 and 73–76; and Sandra Beth Lewenson, *Taking Charge: Nursing, Suffrage, and Feminism in America, 1873–1920* (New York: Garland, 1993), 17–24.

13. The first nursing schools were established in 1873; prior to this time "nurses" did not have to have any formalized training. Reverby, *Ordered to Care*, 61.

14. Schultz, "Inhospitable Hospital," 364–65.

15. According to Schultz, women's presence in hospitals "created a front where gender, class, and racial identities became themselves sites of conflict." Schultz, *Women at the Front*, 3; and Leonard, *Yankee Women*, introduction and p. 200.

16. The specification that Dix alone could approve the hiring of any nurse led to resentment on the part of many military surgeons (males) who saw Dix's appointment as an affront to their military authority. Further, surgeons, who believed that many of Dix's nurses lacked the submissive qualities they felt necessary to maintaining medical and military hierarchies, did not always accept her choice of nurses. Dix's authority to appoint nurses was stripped by 1863, when the surgeon general gave surgeons the ability to appoint and hire their own nurses. Leonard, *Yankee Women*, 6–7 and 16–18.

17. Ibid., 16–17; Schultz, "Inhospitable Hospital," 369.

18. According to Schultz, because of prejudice, "most African American women were given the jobs of cooking and washing . . . whereas higher prestige jobs [nurse and matron] were reserved for whites." Schultz, *Women at the Front*, 21–22.

19. Schultz further points out that the female workforce was composed of both white and black women under the auspices of hospital worker, even if they did not have the official title of nurse; therefore, scholars must realize that the female workforce (Union and Confederate, black and white) was at least twice the size most often documented. *Women at the Front*, 5.

20. Pay discrepancies existed between black and white women. Most of the women who had access to pay worked for Dix. Black women typically earned ten dollars per month as nurses, white women twelve dollars. Schultz, *Women at the Front*, 7; see also Major Julia C. Stimson and Ethel C. S. Thompson, "Women Nurses with the Union Forces during the Civil War," *Military Surgeon* (January–February 1928): 227.

21. Some upper-class and upper-middle-class women were reluctant to take pay for what they viewed was a feminine obligation. Schultz, *Women at the Front*, 42–43.

22. There are contradictory estimates on the numbers of women who served as nurses. Union numbers suggest roughly thirty-two hundred women served as nurses; however, this does not take into account black women, for example, who served as nurses while hired as cooks and washers. Safe estimates, according to historian Jane Schultz, double that number, but she suggests also that the number may be closer to twenty thousand. Jeanne Holm, *Women in the Military: An Unfinished Revolution* (Novato, Calif.: Presidio, 1992), 13–14; and Schultz, *Women at the Front*, 5.

23. Schultz, *Women at the Front*, 173.

24. From the fourth century through the fifteenth century, Christian (religious) hospitals and other institutions for the sick flourished in areas throughout Europe. Men within religious orders played a major role in their expansion and in service as nurses. For example, for their work with the sick, the Catholic Church canonized St. Ephrem and St. Basil the Great. Chad E. O'Lynn and Russell E. Tranbarger, eds., *Men in Nursing: History, Challenges, and Opportunity* (New York: Springer, 2007), 10–11; and Joan Lane, *A Social History of Medicine: Health, Healing, and Disease in England, 1750–1950* (London: Routledge, 2001), introduction.

25. Through the 1720s, midwives in England were required to procure a "bishop's license" to practice. So, although sex segregation often divided the work that men and women performed, men still controlled whether a women could practice as a midwife. Lane, *Social History of Medicine*, 120–26.

26. These three orders were dedicated to the Holy Spirit, to the care of the sick during the Great Plague, and to providing comfort to those who were dying. Not all of these orders began as religious orders, but many developed into or became closely associated with religious orders. The Brotherhood of Santo Spirito gained favor from Pope Innocent III in 1204, and by 1476 Pope Sixtus IV declared that only members

of the clergy could be leaders of the group. Similarly, the Alexian Brothers, although founded in the twelfth century, were by the fifteenth century a religious community. Finally, the Brothers of the Happy Death order was founded by laymen who later became priests. O'Lynn and Tranbarger, *Men in Nursing*, 18–21.

27. Ibid.

28. Four nursing orders have received the most attention from nursing scholars. These orders include the Knights Hospitallers of St. John of Jerusalem, the Knights of St. Lazarus, the Templar Knights, and the Teutonic Knights. All four orders originally founded hospitals that treated the poor, sick pilgrims, or wounded soldiers; however, as the orders evolved, their dedication to nursing and military pursuits grew as well. The Templars and the Teutonic Knights, for example, eventually devoted more of their time and energy to military activities during the twelfth and thirteenth centuries. The Hospitallers, in contrast, remained dedicated to their hospital and nursing, although they did take up arms at various points of their existence. Finally, the Knights of St. Lazarus abandoned their hospital mission altogether at the end of the thirteenth century and dedicated themselves fully to military activities until they ceased to exist during the French Revolution. Ibid., 13–18.

29. Sarah Gamp is a character in Charles Dickens's *Martin Chuzzlewit*. She was a trained nurse who was often drunk and perhaps mentally unstable. Ibid., 18–20; Carolyn Mackintosh, "A Historical Study of Men in Nursing," *Journal of Advanced Nursing* 26, no. 2 (1997): 233; and Joan Evans, "Male Nurses: A Historical and Feminist Perspective," *Journal of Advanced Nursing* 47, no. 3 (2004): 322.

30. O'Lynn and Tranbarger, *Men in Nursing*, 21–24.

31. Nightingale's nurses successfully reversed the mortality rate for British soldiers by instituting basic sanitation and rigorous monitoring of patients' care and diet. Kalisch and Kalisch, *Advance of American Nursing*, 32–36.

32. Male soldiers served as nurses prior to this, but on a purely voluntary basis and usually because of their own recuperation in the hospital. In other words, nursing was an untrained, temporary activity for them. Mary T. Sarnecky, *A History of the U.S. Army Nurse Corps*, Studies in Health, Illness, and Caregiving (Philadelphia: University of Pennsylvania Press, 1999), 12; "The Army Hospital Corps," *Medical News* (January 28, 1888): 104.

33. Harvey E. Brown, *The Medical Department of the United States Army from 1775–1873* (Washington, D.C.: Surgeon General's Office, 1873); and Sarnecky, *History*, 12.

34. Stimson and Thompson, "Women Nurses," 227; and Schultz, *Women at the Front*, 7.

35. Lewenson, *Taking Charge*, 24.

36. The three training schools opened in the United States in 1873 were Bellevue Training School for Nurses in New York City, Connecticut Training School for Nurses in New Haven, and Boston Training School for Nurses in Massachusetts. White philanthropic activist women backed all. Ibid., 21–25.

37. In 1889, the Johns Hopkins School of Nursing was the first school open in the United States with direct consultation from Florence Nightingale.

38. At late as 1958, LeRoy Craig encouraged male nurses to be athletic and physically fit as part of their training. Mackintosh, "Historical Study," 233; Evans, "Male Nurses"; Bruce P. Mericle, "The Male as Psychiatric Nurse," *Journal of Psychosocial Nursing* 21, no. 11 (1983): 28–34; R. D. Rider, "Letters to the Editor," *American Journal of Nursing* 3, no. 7 (April 1903): 582–83; and Augustana Nurse, "Letters to the Editor," *American Journal of Nursing*, 3, no. 9 (June 1903): 742.

39. Nona Y. Glazer, "'Between a Rock and a Hard Place': Women's Professional Organizations in Nursing and Class, Racial, and Ethnic Inequalities," *Gender and Society* 5, no. 3 (September 1991): 351–72.

40. There are several schools that can be discussed here; for brevity, I have kept the discussion to the four most well known.

41. Mericle, "Male as Psychiatric Nurse," 30–31.

42. O'Lynn and Tranbarger, *Men in Nursing*, 44–46.

43. Ibid., 45.

44. There is no mention about the race of the students attending these institutions; however, in keeping with race segregation of the period, it is safe to assume that most students were white men. Most schools of nursing dedicated to educating African Americans do not mention black males. Instead, information about the black male medical professionals most often focused on black male doctors. This is worth noting because the American Nurses' Association census reported 127 black graduate male nurses and nurse students in the United States in 1940. See Appendix C herewith and also Vanessa Northington Gamble, *Making a Place for Ourselves: The Black Hospital Movement, 1920–1945* (New York: Oxford University Press, 1995), 44.

45. While male nurses make up fewer than 10 percent of the nursing population in 2012, they represent nearly 45 percent of nurse anesthetists. "Certified Registered Nurse Anesthetists at a Glance," available at http://www.aana.com/ceandeducation/becomeacrna/Pages/Nurse-Anesthetists-at-a-Glance.aspx (accessed on July 17, 2012).

46. Tillman E. Barrington, interviewed by Cindy Houser, University of North Texas Oral History Project 989 (May 22, 1992), 2.

47. Opposition to the professionalization of nursing varied for much the same reason the employment of female nurses did during the Civil War. Paternalistic physicians and the medical profession worried about loss of control over this part of the medical field. Supporters of nurse professionalization pointed to the hierarchical nature of nurse training that would ensure that while nurses mastered their field within the medical profession, they would always be placed as an assistant to doctors. Wood, "Nurse and the Medical Man," 279–81; and "Organized Opposition," in *AJN* "Editorial Comments," 5.

48. McGee asked the wife of the chief of surgery at Freedman's Hospital in Washington, D.C., to work as a nurse because she had already had yellow fever. She also asked for help in securing the service of other African American nurses who were

immune to yellow fever. Additionally, McGee contracted with about 250 nuns. There is also some indication that about fifteen male nurses served as contract workers; however, according to Army Nurse Corps history, these men were not under the jurisdiction of McGee but worked directly with doctors. M. Elizabeth Carnegie, *The Path We Tread: Blacks in Nursing 1854–1990* (New York: National League for Nursing Press, 1991), 12–15; Sarnecky, *History*, 29–30; Reverby, *Ordered to Care*, 60–62; Linda Grant De Pauw, *Battle Cries and Lullabies: Women in War from Prehistory to the Present* (Norman: University of Oklahoma Press, 1998): 200–204.

49. The ANC was not a permanent part of the Medical Department; nurses contracted during the Spanish-American War included women of various backgrounds, and men. It was not until nursing became an official entity within the army that the ANC became almost uniformly homogenous with regard to sex and race. Sarnecky, *History*, 31 and 36; and De Pauw, *Battle Cries and Lullabies*, 202–3.

50. Holm, *Women in the Military*, 8–9; and Sarnecky, *History*, 36–37, 42, 50.

51. As a quasi-military auxiliary with the U.S. Army, female nurses received no military rank, equivalent pay, or retirement and veterans' benefits.

52. The Nurses Associated Alumnae of the United States and Canada was founded in 1896 as the precursor to the American Nurses' Association.

53. Pocklington, *Heritage of Leadership*, 13–17.

54. Sarnecky, *History*, 50–53 and 29–31.

55. Most Southern nursing schools banned black women, while those in the North imposed strict quotas on their enrollment. Mary Mahoney, graduate of the New England Hospital for Women and Children in 1878, was the first African American woman to complete a nursing program. It was not until the 1890s that nurse training schools for African American women began to open with any regularity. Most of these schools were founded by black physicians in conjunction with hospital schools. Reverby, *Ordered to Care*; Hine, *Black Women in White*; and Carnegie, *Path We Tread*, 19–20.

56. Before 1916 a small group of African American nurses did join the American Nurses' Association. However, a change in the bylaws in 1916 meant that African American nurses were denied access to the most prominent national nursing association. As a result, they had difficulty enrolling with American Red Cross and joining ANC.

57. Martha Franklin, a graduate of the Woman's Hospital in Philadelphia, surveyed black nurses across the country over a two-year period with the idea of forming a national organization for black nurses. She and fifty-one other graduate nurses met in New York in 1908 and founded the National Association of Colored Graduate Nurses. Franklin became the first president of the organization. "A Salute to Democracy in Nursing at Mid-Century," *National Association of Colored Graduate Nurses Records, 1908–1951*, 1984, New York Public Library, Schomburg Center for Research in Black Culture, reel 2.

58. "A Salute to Democracy in Nursing," 6–10.

59. Refer to Sarnecky, *History*, 50–53 and 29–31, regarding changes in membership requirements for the ANA.

60. Darlene Clark Hine, "The Call That Never Came: Black Women Nurses and World War I; An Historical Note," *Indiana Military History Journal* (January 1983): 23–24.

61. The Red Cross classified nurses into the first, second, and third reserves by World War II. These classifications appeared to be based on their qualifications and the needs of the nurse corps, but discrimination also played a role in classification. Almost all African American female nurses classified as second or third reserve. This system became one focus of the integration campaign by African American nurses.

62. During World War I, Aileen Cole Stewart was one of eighteen Negro nurses to serve as a Red Cross Nurse and with the ANC during World War I. Aileen Cole Stewart, "Ready to Serve," *American Journal of Nursing* 63 (September 1963): 85–87; Hine, *Black Women in White*, 102–3 and 167; and Sarnecky, *History*, 127.

63. Chad Williams, *Torchbearers of Democracy: African American Soldiers in the World War I Era* (Chapel Hill: University of North Carolina Press, 2010), introduction; Adriane Lentz-Smith, *Freedom Struggles: African Americans and World War I* (Cambridge, Mass.: Harvard University Press, 2009); and Hine, "Call That Never Came," 24.

64. National Association for the Advancement of Colored People, hereinafter known as NAACP. Timothy B. Tyson, *Radio Free Dixie: Robert F. Williams and the Roots of Black Power* (Chapel Hill: University of North Carolina Press, 1999), 26–30; and W. Stuart Towns, ed., *We Want Our Freedom: Rhetoric of the Civil Rights Movement* (New York: Praeger, 2000).

Chapter 2. "The Negro Nurse—A Citizen Fighting for Democracy"

1. In addition to the Service Men's Wives, other organizations that participated in the campaign included the National Sweethearts of Servicemen, the Nurses' Local Union, and the National Council of Negro Women. National Archives and Records Administration, College Park, Md., [hereinafter NARA], RG 52, box 6.

2. There were other minority female nurses who wished to join the ANC at the same time; however, their numbers were substantially smaller, and as a group they were less organized than African American female nurses. For example, according to the ANC, four Japanese American and fourteen Puerto Rican women served as nurses. Mary Standlee and Col. Florence Blanchfield, unpublished manuscript [1950?], "The Appointment of Racial Minorities in the ANC," Army Nurse Corps Archives, Office of the Surgeon General [hereinafter as ANCA, OSG], Falls Church, Va., box 108.

3. Historians Robert Korstad and Martha Biondi characterize the period between the Great Depression and the mid-1940s as one of "civil rights unionism" and the "Black Popular Front," respectively, and as a precursor to the "modern" civil rights movement of the postwar period. Here, I argue for the necessity of viewing the civil

rights movement as one long, continuous movement, as put forth in Jacquelyn Dowd Hall's "The Long Civil Rights Movement." Further, while the terms "modern" and "classical" are often used interchangeably to discuss the movement after 1954, I will be using "modern" to discuss and define the long civil rights movement from the early decades of the twentieth century through the mid-1960s and will reserve the term "classical" for the period that has become quintessentially defined as the civil rights movement, 1954–1965. Jacquelyn Dowd Hall, "The Long Civil Rights Movement and the Political Uses of the Past," *Journal of American History* 91, no. 4 (March 2005): 1233–63; Robert Rodgers Korstad, *Civil Rights Unionism: Tobacco Workers and the Struggle for Democracy in the Mid-Twentieth-Century South* (Chapel Hill: University of North Carolina Press, 2003); and Martha Biondi, *To Stand and Fight: The Struggle for Civil Rights in Postwar New York City* (Cambridge, Mass.: Harvard University Press, 2003).

4. Nancy MacLean defines the "culture of exclusion" as one that keeps racism and discrimination so much a part of daily relationships that it is overlooked as normative. Nancy MacLean, *Freedom Is Not Enough: The Opening of the American Workplace* (Cambridge, Mass.: Harvard University Press, 2006), 22.

5. Ibid., 4; Hall, "Long Civil Rights Movement," 1245–46.

6. Maj. Julia O. Flikke, October 2, 1940, Records of the National Association of Colored Graduate Nurses, 1908–1951, reel 2.

7. African American female nurses were not the only racial minorities who attempted to join the ANC. According to an unpublished manuscript on the use of racial minorities in the ANC during World War II, by the end of the war, only a small number of Japanese Americans and Puerto Ricans served with the nurse corps. The secretary of war, however, "defined a clear-cut policy which protected their appointment." Japanese-American women who wished to serve could only do so under the following conditions: be citizens of the United States and cleared by the Provost Marshall General's Office as to loyalty; found to be professionally and physically qualified, the latter qualification being determined by the standard of the WACs; acquiescent to the direction of the surgeon general in their assignment to duty. Due to their small numbers and the worry that their presence—in the case of Japanese Americans—might "antagonize military patients," there were few who served during the war. Standlee and Blanchfield, "Appointment of Racial Minorities," 31–34.

8. Pearl McIver, Senior Nursing Consultant, U.S. Public Service for National Negro Health Week, April 1943, "Negro Nurses and the War Effort," Mabel K. Staupers Papers, Moorland-Spingarn Research Center, Howard University, Washington, D.C. [hereinafter MSRC], box 96-2.

9. Besides the Army Nurse Corps, established by Congress in 1901, the U.S. Navy also had its own nurse corps that was established by an act of Congress in 1908.

10. In a letter to the *Pittsburgh Courier*, James G. Thompson called on African Americans to fight a "Double V" campaign of their own. Black newspapers supported Thompson's suggestion of fighting for victory over fascism abroad and victory over

discrimination at home by creating the movement in 1942. *National News Bulletin* 16, no. 33 (August 1942).

11. Estelle Massey Osborne, "Status and Contribution of the Negro Nurse," *Journal of Negro Education* 18 (1949): 364.

12. The professionalization of nursing was an ongoing process that evolved over much of the twentieth century. The first nursing schools opened in 1873. Those in the South, however, banned black women, while those in the North imposed strict quotas on their attendance. It was not until the 1890s that nurse training schools for African American women began to open with any regularity. A partnership between black physicians and hospital schools founded most of these schools. Reverby, *Ordered to Care*; and Hine, *Black Women in White*.

13. According to Lucy E. Salyer, during World War I "military service became the ultimate test of a man's Americanness and a compelling organizing principle of U.S. citizenship policy." While Salyer is explicitly exploring the use of military service by non-U.S. citizens to argue for citizenship rights, she does point to the historic contradictions of war, military participation, and citizenship definitions in U.S. history. That is, regardless of demonstrating loyalty to the nation through military service, racialized ideals of citizenship remained intact through the mid-twentieth century, thus hindering citizenship benefits from even race minorities who were already citizens and who participated in defending the United States. Lucy E. Salyer, "Baptism by Fire: Race, Military Service, and U.S. Citizenship Policy, 1918–1935," *Journal of American History* 91, no. 3 (December 2004): 847–76; and Gary Gerstle, *American Crucible: Race and Nation in the Twentieth Century* (Princeton, N.J.: Princeton University Press, 2001).

14. Sarnecky, *History*, 50.

15. There is evidence of male nurses challenging this policy as early as World War I. The next chapter will address male nurses exclusively. For more information on male nurses and military service, see O'Lynn and Tranbarger, *Men in Nursing*.

16. Reverby, *Ordered to Care*, 199–207.

17. The evolution of nursing into a professional extension of "women's natural work" did not begin until after the Civil War. After the success of this experience and participation in the War of 1898, these female nurses lobbied Congress to establish a permanent Nurse Corps. Ibid., chapter 1.

18. Appointment to the ANC was different from "induction" into the U.S. military. Male soldiers were inducted into the military upon enlistment in a service branch. The surgeon general approved women to serve in the U.S. Army Nurse Corps; women did not just enlist. This was one way to avoid the possibility of women seeking certain benefits, such as retirement at highest rank. Nurses' rank was "relative" until the middle of World War II, which meant that their rank was comparable to those ranks attached to men in the permanent army. However, their treatment within the officers' corps and the benefits available to them differed from men of similar rank. Sarnecky, *History*, 29–31 and 50–53; and "Male Nurse Demands Equal Rights for Men," newspaper clipping (May 1944), ANCA, OSG, box 110.

19. During World War I, Aileen Cole Stewart served with the American Red Cross and the ANC. Her story is a primary example of the availability and desire of African Americans to serve their country. All African American nurses who eventually served in the ANC during World War I came from the Red Cross. Aileen Cole Stewart, "Ready to Serve," *American Journal of Nursing* 63 (September 1963): 85–87.

20. Historians Chad Williams and Adriane Lentz-Smith argue that black participation during World War I radicalized an entire generation of African American activists. A. Phillip Randolph's work with the Brotherhood of Sleeping Car Porters is just one example of the rise of black militancy in the interwar period. Williams, *Torchbearers of Democracy*; Lentz-Smith, *Freedom Struggles*.

21. Gamble, *Making a Place.*

22. The journal began in 1932 at Howard University. In 1937 (vol. 6, no. 3) and again in 1949 (vol. 18, no. 3), the *Journal of Negro Education* dedicated their summer issues to the health status and health education of Negroes in the United States. The contributors focused not only on mortality and sickness rates but also on access to medical care and facilities, and the training and supply of medical professionals. Louis I. Dublin, "The Problems of Negro Health as Revealed by Vital Statistics," *Journal of Negro Education* 18, no. 3 (Summer 1949): 209.

23. Estelle Massey Riddle, "The Education of the Negro Nurse," as quoted in Alma C. Haupt, "A Pioneer in Negro Nursing," *American Journal of Nursing* 35, no. 9 (September 1935): 859.

24. On a 1937 list of hospitals that employed and/or trained black nurses, only two dozen of the roughly 115 hospitals had nursing schools registered with the State Board of Nurse Examiners. Estelle Massey Riddle, "Sources of Supply of Negro Health Personnel, Section C: Nurses," *Journal of Negro Education* 6, no. 3 (1937): 484–86.

25. A 1937 table in Riddle, "Sources of Supply," focused on the distribution of Negro nurses in hospitals that "employed, trained, or both," indicated only three mixed hospitals: Charity Hospital in New Orleans; Jersey City Hospital in Jersey City, N.J.; and City Hospital in Buffalo, N.Y. On the growth of the black hospital movement, see Gamble, *Making a Place.*

26. Numa P. G. Adams, "Sources of Supply of Negro Health Personnel, Section A: Physicians," *Journal of Negro Education* 6, no. 3 (1937): 468; see also Smith, *Sick and Tired.*

27. Riddle, "Sources of Supply," 483–92.

28. American Nurses' Association, "ANA Committees Concerned with the Status of Colored Graduate Nurses," [1936?] American Nurses' Association Collection, Headquarters Files, Silver Spring, Md.

29. Patricia D'Antonio, *American Nursing: A History of Knowledge, Authority, and the Meaning of Work* (Baltimore, Md.: Johns Hopkins University Press, 2010), 127–30.

30. Esther Lucile Brown, *Nursing for the Future: A Report Prepared for the National Nursing Council* (New York: Sage, 1948), 7.

31. Black nurses began to retaliate in the early 1930s as they attempted to redefine the status and place of African American female nurses within the larger nursing

establishment and called for better educational opportunities and images of nurses. Estelle Massey Riddle, "What Is a Nurse?" *Opportunity* 12, no. 2 (February 1934): 52–53.

32. Historian Stephanie Shaw discussed the high status bestowed by the community on African American nurses. Stephanie Shaw, *What a Women Ought to Be and Do: Black Professional Women Workers During the Jim Crow Era* (Chicago: University of Chicago Press, 1996), 3 and 150.

33. Riddle, "Education," 859.

34. Most state and national nursing associations restricted membership by race, with few exceptions. Therefore, most nonwhite nurses had difficulty attaining membership in the premier professional nursing organization, the American Nurses' Association. The National Organization of Public Health Nurses eventually accepted black nurses through their membership in the NACGN. By the 1930s three types of nurses existed: the private-duty nurse, the largest proportion of nurses, also known as the "graduate or trained nurse"; the hospital-staff nurse, often student or untrained nurses doing most of the general work in hospitals; and the public health nurse, the smallest group of trained nurses, working with volunteer or government-sponsored public health programs servicing the poor and working class. The focus of professional organizations and their willingness to welcome and include minority nurses in their organizations becomes most apparent when examining class status and the educational backgrounds of their members. For example, the American Nurses' Association consisted mainly of white, private-duty nurses, trained at many of the elite nursing institutions in the country. In contrast, staff nurses were often untrained nurses, and a majority of black nurses worked as public health nurses, who, although trained, were often less educated. As public health nursing declined and staff nursing attracted trained nurses in the 1930s, these groups became an economic threat to elite-trained nurses.

35. Hine, *Black Women in White*, 108–11.

36. Ibid., 112.

37. Jane Van De Vrede, "Report of Committee on Joint Relations with the National Association of Colored Graduate Nurses," April 15, 1934, American Nurses' Association Collection, Headquarters Files, Silver Spring, Md.; Hine, *Black Women in White*, 112–13.

38. The Rosenwald Fund was established in 1917 by wealthy American clothier Julius Rosenwald for the "well-being of mankind." Rosenwald became interested in social issues, especially the education of African Americans. The fund began with Rosenwald's donation to Booker T. Washington that provided assistance to the educational endeavors of African Americans. By 1917 the fund became its own entity, providing support for a variety of African American and Jewish social causes. This mission eventually grew to include black healthcare and black nurses, and, in the 1930s, the National Association of Colored Graduate Nurses. The fund donated $2,150 to the General Budget of the NACGN. Edwin Embree and Julia Waxman, *Investment*

in the People: The Story of the Julius Rosenwald Fund (New York: Harper, 1949), Appendix D, p. 272; Emily W. Bennett, "The Work of a Rosenwald Nurse," *Public Health Nurse* 23 (March 1931): 119–20; Mabel K. Staupers, *No Time for Prejudice: A Story of the Integrations of Negroes in Nursing in the United States* (New York: Macmillan, 1961), 31–32.

39. Examples of some of the race-advocacy groups that Riddle and Staupers encouraged participation in were the NAACP and the National Urban League. The NACGN was also instrumental in the founding of the National Council of Negro Women. Staupers, *No Time for Prejudice*, 34–46; and Hine, *Black Women in White*, 126.

40. Hine, *Black Women in White*, 121.

41. Homer G. Phillips was, until 1936, City Hospital #2 in St. Louis, Missouri. It was a hospital for black patients in the area and was one of the few hospitals approved to provide internships for black doctors and to train black nurses. Adams, "Sources of Supply of Negro Health Personnel, Section A: Physicians," 474; and Riddle, "Sources of Supply," 485.

42. Riddle's actual score was a 93.3 percent on her Missouri State Board Examination, purportedly the highest achieved at that point in history by a black woman. Hine, *Black Women in White*, 117–19.

43. Ibid., 118.

44. Haupt, "Pioneer in Negro Nursing," 857–58; and Hine, *Black Women in White*, 117–19.

45. The word "white" was added to the quote for clarification in order to give the reader a sense of who the public was. Ibid., 117–19.

46. The Booker T. Washington Sanitarium was one of the first facilities that permitted black physicians to treat patients. Ibid., 119.

47. Biographical data, Mabel K. Staupers Papers, MSRC, folder 1; Hine, *Black Women in White*, 118–21.

48. Originally, the NACGN had organized the country into six regions but consolidated them into four by 1937. Each region had elected officers who acted as intermediaries between nurses and the community in their region and between the region and the association's headquarters in New York. Staupers, *No Time for Prejudice*, 29–53; and Hine, *Black Women in White*, 124–26. See also the list of conferences in February 1944, and in the correspondence between Staupers and Colonel Blanchfield, which reveal the need to have an army nurse attending as part of a recruitment campaign, ANCA, OSG, box 108.

49. Staupers, *No Time for Prejudice*, 34.

50. Hine, *Black Women in White*, 126–27; and Staupers, *No Time for Prejudice*, 30–35.

51. Walter White to Mabel K. Staupers, December 16, 1942, Records of the National Association for the Advancement of Colored People, part 15: Segregation and Discrimination: Complaints and Responses, 1940–1955, series B, reel 9, frame 295; see also frames: 296 and 298. Frame 338 is a letter from Carrie F. Walker to Walter

White, October 7, 1942, asking for assistance on the transfer and mistreatment of twenty black nurses from a veterans' facility in Tuskegee.

52. Records, NAACP, part 15, series B, reel 9, frame 366, and part 18, series B, reel 8, frames 190–91, 202–04, and 209–11.

53. "Attacks 'Snoopervision' at Nurses Conference," *Chicago Defender*, March 18, 1939.

54. *National News Bulletin* 16, no. 33 (August 1942).

55. Repeated letters to and meetings with representatives from the Red Cross, the American Nurses' Association, and the Army Nurse Corps between 1920 and 1940 attest to the fact that the black nurses were diligent in their pursuit for integration and inclusion in these organizations. "ANA Committee Concerned with the Status of Colored Graduate Nurses," [1936] Meeting of ANA Board of Directors, American Nurses' Association Collection, Headquarters Files, Silver Spring, Md.; and Stewart, "Ready to Serve."

56. Secretary to Dr. Louis Wright to Ruth L. Roberts, September 25 and October 2, 1940, Records, NAACP, part 15, series B, reel 9, frames 165–67.

57. Ibid.; see also American Nurses' Association, "Joint Conference," October 28, 1940, American Nurses' Association Collection, Howard Gotlieb Archival Research Center, Boston University [hereinafter as HGARC], box 329.

58. Franklin Delano Roosevelt to Walter White, October 25, 1940, Franklin D. Roosevelt Papers, Official Files 93, container 3, folder "Colored Matters," Franklin Delano Roosevelt Archives, Hyde Park, N.Y., as quoted in Hine, *Black Women in White*, 167.

59. "Nurses Rally Here to Fight Color Quotas," *Chicago Defender*, March 13, 1943.

60. Staupers, *No Time for Prejudice*, 100–105.

61. Wright to Roberts, September 25 and October 2, 1940; Maj. Julia O. Flikke, October 2, 1940, NACGN Records, 1908–1951, reel 1; Hine, *Black Women in White*, 165–66; Records of the Office of the Surgeon General of the United States Army, RG 112, NARA; and Ulysses Lee, *The Employment of Negro Troops* (Washington, D.C.: Office of the Chief of Military History, United States Army, 1966): 83 and 196–97.

62. Staupers, *No Time for Prejudice*, 101. The idea for A. Philip Randolph's March on Washington Movement was only in its infancy in late 1940, as Randolph, Walter White of the NAACP, and T. Arnold Hill of the National Urban League pushed the president to take a firm stand to support African American participation in war mobilization. The plans quickly became a reality once it was apparent that the status quo would be maintained.

63. The Red Cross was the procurement organization for the Army Nurse Corps and had been since the organization's founding in 1901. All nurses who wished to join the ANC first registered with the Red Cross and were ranked based on a series of qualifications. Flikke, October 2, 1940.

64. Mabel K. Staupers to President Franklin D. Roosevelt, October 26, 1940, ANCA, OSG, Falls Church, Va., box 108; "Status of the Negro Nurse in the Army Nursing

Corps," n.d., Records, NAACP, part 9: Discrimination in the U.S. Armed Forces, 1918–1955, series A, reel 12, frame 730.

65. Staupers to President Roosevelt, October 26, 1940.

66. Surgeon General's Office (S.G.O.) to Mabel K. Staupers, October 31, 1940, ANCA, OSG, box 108.

67. Chief of Staff to Secretary of War, December 1, 1941, as quoted in Ulysses Lee's *The Employment of Negro Troops* (Washington, D.C.: Office of the Chief of Military History, 1966), 140.

68. James Magee to Mary Beard, April 8, 1941, NARA, RG 112.

69. Chief of Staff to Secretary of War, December 1, 1941, 140–41.

70. "Status of the Negro Nurse," NAACP; Stewart, "Ready to Serve."

71. According to this 1927 letter, there were only four black regiments in the army; one at each of the following locations: Fort Riley, Kansas; Fort Benning, Georgia; Fort Hauchuca and Nogales, Arizona. Darnall, C.R., Colonel to Honorable Andrew L. Somers, June 6, 1927, ANCA, OSG, box 108.

72. Ibid.

73. "Army's McGee Bared as Jim Crow Exponent," *Chicago Defender*, February 7, 1942.

74. "Status of the Negro Nurse."

75. Holding tight to the opinion that segregation was a "law of nature," Senator Theodore Bilbo of Mississippi was a prolific writer on what he viewed as the proper role of African Americans in the United States. He feared that the military's use of African Americans would lead them to believe that they were socially equal to whites, and he warned that the military must maintain segregation at all cost or the post-war period would be marked by racial conflict. Senator Theodore Bilbo to General Dwight D. Eisenhower, December 15, 1945, NARA, RG 165, box 189.

76. "Status of the Negro Nurse."

77. As quoted in Philip A. Kalisch and Beatrice J. Kalisch, *The Advance of American Nursing* (Philadelphia: Lippincott, 1995): 349.

78. In October 1940, the surgeon general issued the Army's "plan for the use of colored personnel," which first stipulated that no provisions were made for the employment of African American nurses, and then only for the limited use of African Americans nurses in areas where "colored troops dominated." Flikke, October 2, 1940; Maj. Julia O. Flikke to Mabel K. Staupers, December 10, 1941, NACGN Records, 1908–1951, reel 2; Lee, *Employment of Negro Troops*, 196–97.

79. "Negro Nurses to Serve in the U.S. Army," *Chicago Defender*, February 8, 1941.

80. These are just two examples of the headlines that continued to grace the pages of the black press. "Appeal for Integration Is Ignored," *Chicago Defender*, March 21, 1942, and "Army Edict Bars Nurses," *Chicago Defender*, March 13, 1943.

81. The surgeon general issued the army's "plan for the use of colored personnel," which stipulated that there were no provisions in "Army regulations for the appointment of Negro nurses in the Nurse Corps," and the army would use African American

nurses only in areas where "colored troops dominated." Flikke to Staupers, December 10, 1941.

82. Kirk, SG to Representative Robert Crosser, November 20, 1943, ANCA, OSG, box 108.

83. Lt. Col. Ida W. Danielson to Miss Carolyn E. Dillon, October 13, 1943, reprinted in: *PM*, October 24, 1943; and "African American Nurses—End of Month."

84. Ruth Murray, "Army and Navy Need 60,000, but Stick to Color Line," *PM*, October 24, 1943.

85. Frank A. Young, "Claim War Effort Lacks Total Support," *Chicago Defender*, January 17, 1942.

86. Mabel K. Staupers to Mary Beard, January 4, 1941, Mabel K. Staupers Papers, MSRC, box 96-1, folder 3.

87. Young, "Claim War Effort."

88. Al Smith, "U.S. Answers Nurse Charge," *Chicago Defender*, April 8, 1944; "Jim Crow Blacks Army Call for Needed Nurses," *Chicago Defender*, December 30, 1944; "Negro Nurses Hit Jim Crow Policy of Army, Navy," *Chicago Defender*, December 30, 1944.

89. Public Health Service, *The United States Cadet Nurse Corps and Other Federal Nursing Training Programs 1943–48* (Washington, D.C.: Government Printing Office, 1950), 1.

90. In the early summer of 1943, Congress passed H.R. 2664, the Nurse Training Act. President Roosevelt signed the act on June 15, 1943, and it became Public Law 74 on July 1, 1943. Ibid., 30.

91. Ibid., 31 and 49.

92. Elmira B. Wickenden, R.N., "The National Nursing Council Reports," *American Journal of Nursing* 43, no. 9 (September 1943): 807.

93. The National Nursing Council for War Service, "Institute: The Negro Nurse and the War," February 15, 1943, American Nurses' Association Collection, HGARC, box 228.

94. See Appendix A herewith (*Facts about Negro Nurses and the War*, prepared by the National Association of Colored Graduate Nurses and the National Nursing Council for War Service); and Public Health Service, *The United States Cadet Nurse Corps and Other Federal Nursing Training Programs 1943–48*, 49.

95. National Association of Colored Graduate Nurses and the National Nursing Council for War Service, February 21, 1945, *Facts about Negro Nurses and the War* (New York: NACGN and NNCWS Headquarters, 1945), ANCA, OSG, box 108.

96. Black nurses were eventually stationed, at various points in the war, in Liberia, New Guinea, the United Kingdom, and Scotland, among others.

97. *Facts about Negro Nurses and the War*, February 21, 1945.

98. The National Nursing Council for War Service (NNCWS) was originally the Nursing Council on National Defense but in 1943 changed its name. The council formed in the summer of 1940 with representation from the ANA, National League

of Nursing Education, and the National Organization for Public Health Nursing; af-
filiated members included the Red Cross and NACGN. See Standlee and Blanchfield,
"Appointment of Racial Minorities."

99. See Appendix A herewith; NACGN and NNCWS, *Facts about Negro Nurses*.

100. In early 1944 Walter White toured the ETO (European Theater of Operations)
to observe and make recommendations on race relations. This tour, supported by the
U.S. Army, reported that the "American High Command" recognized the "existence
of the problem" and was taking "affirmative steps towards its correction." White
was encouraged by steps meant to reduce race discrimination, including issuing
directives about the treatment of all American soldiers and educating white soldiers
about their behavior toward black soldiers. He made his own recommendations on
how to help increase black morale and lessen race tensions. The most important was
the increased training of black officers and use of black combat troops. This report
was filed with the office of the secretary of war and given to General Eisenhower
and General Lee and Ambassador John G. Winant (the U.S. ambassador to Great
Britain). Walter White, "Observations and Recommendations of Walter White on
Racial Relations in the ETO," February 11, 1944, NARA, RG 107, box 447.

101. Sarnecky, *History*, 271.

102. Every few months between 1943 and 1945 procurement numbers change from
forty thousand to fifty thousand and then back to forty thousand, and, by late 1944,
sixty thousand. Major Edna B. Groppe, "Statement made at the public hearing before
the House Military Affairs Committee on February 14, 1945," *American Journal of
Nursing* 45 (March 1945): 175; "Recruitment material," American Nurses' Association
Collection, HGARC, box 228.

103. "Seek 8,500 More Nurses," *New York Times*, July 18, 1944.

104. Staupers, "Negro Nurses Would Serve," *New York Times*, December 19, 1944;
"Suggests Negro Nurses," *New York Times*, January 12, 1945; "Would Use Negro
Nurses," *New York Times*, January 21, 1945; and Ramona Lowe, "Army Lifts Quota
Ban on Nurses," *Chicago Defender*, July 15, 1944.

105. Smith, "U.S. Answers Nurse Charge."

106. Ibid.

107. Fears about lesbians and unfeminine women led the military to have strict
policies concerning the appearance and behaviors of women in uniform during
World War II. Leisa Meyer, *Creating G.I. Jane: Sexuality and Power in the Women's
Army Corps During World War II* (New York: Columbia University Press, 1998).

108. The cartoon was part of a series of cartoons created by Melvin Tapley that
depicted racism and race relations in the United States. On military nurses, Tapley
published two cartoons, commenting on the Army Nurse Corps and Navy Nurse
Corps. Melvin Tapley, "Glad to See You . . . Now!" *New York Amsterdam News*, July
22, 1944; "Army Lifts Ban on Negro Nurses," *PM*, July 12, 1944.

109. Lowe, "Army Lifts Quota Ban"; Truman Gibson (aide to Sec. of War) to Mabel
K. Staupers, July 1944, NACGN Records, 1908–1951.

110. Units of African American nurses arrived in Liberia and the South Pacific in 1943 and in England, Scotland, and Burma in 1944. "First Negro Nurses Land at War Front in Scotland," *New York Amsterdam News*, August 26, 1944.

111. These letters express the general experiences of black nurses at two bases in Arizona and are a good indicator of the black nurse experience. At least one black nurse, however, did write to the alumni association at Howard University at the end of the war and explained that at her last station hospital there was no discrimination, she cared for POWs and white GIs, and she received respect from all the personnel. Unknown author, October 29 and November 16, 1944, Mabel K. Staupers Papers, MSRC, box 96-2; and Lt. Lucia A. Rapley to Mr. Nabrit, May 12, 1945, Howard University Men and Women in the Armed Forces, MSRC, box 122-1.

112. "African American Nurses—End of Month."

113. There are some general references to a few cases where there were opportunities for Negro and white nurses serving abroad in integrated settings. Staupers, "Negro Nurses Would Serve," *New York Times*, December 19, 1944; "Negro Nurses Protest Having to Treat Nazis," *Chicago Defender*, November 11, 1944; Edward B. Toles, "Negro Nurses Tend Nazi War Prisoners in Britain," *Chicago Defender*, December 2, 1944.

114. Groppe, "Statement," 175.

115. Smith, "U.S. Answers Nurse Charge."

116. Walter Lippmann, "American Women and Our Wounded Men," *Washington Post*, December 19, 1944.

117. The Selective Service Act of 1940 instituted the first peace-time draft in the history of the United States and called on every able-bodied man to give one year of service to the nation's military; the inclusion of female nurses to that act would call into question the constitutionality of drafting not only females but an exclusive population of women into the service of the United States.

118. Major General Norman Kirk as quoted in "Nurses Face Draft as Casualties Rise," *Stars and Stripes*, January 7, 1945, ANCA, OSG, box 79.

119. "Army Still Is Balky on Using Negro Nurses: Surgeon General Admits Drafting May Be Necessary," *PM*, January 5, 1945.

120. Hine, *Black Women in White*, 178–81.

121. Even First Lady Eleanor Roosevelt, while supportive of an "overall draft of nurses, blasted the Jim-Crow-quota of black nurses." "First Lady Urges End of Ban on Negro Nurses," *Chicago Defender*, January 20, 1945; Hine, *Black Women in White*, 178–81.

122. In an advertisement, Ethel Clyde asks mothers and fathers of American soldiers to telegram their senators to demand Negro nurses be allowed into the army before it was too late to help their sons. Ethel Clyde [telegram] January 30, 1945, Records, NAACP, part 15, series B, reel 9, frame 380.

123. Robert A. Moss to Edith Nourse Rogers, January 18, 1945, Edith Nourse Rogers Papers, Schlesinger Library, Radcliffe Institute, MC 196, box 1, folder 15 [hereinafter SL-RI].

124. Hine, *Black Women in White*, 180–81.

125. National Association of Colored Graduate Nurses, "A Statement from the National Association of Colored Graduate Nurses in Relations to the Extension of the Selective Service Act to Include the Drafting of Nurses," Mabel K. Staupers Papers, MSRC, box 96-2.

126. Although speaking in particular about the situation of African American nurses, Darlene Clark Hine has perhaps the best description of the moment for most Americans. See Hine, *Black Women in White*, 180.

127. The January 20, 1945, declaration by the surgeon general is a little misleading as it pertained to African American nurses. Officially, the army lifted the quotas, or "Jim Crow" ban of black nurses, in early July 1944, but getting African American nurses appointed was still difficult. The January 20, 1945, declaration took the July 1944 end to quotas a step further, ensuring that all qualified female nurses would be accepted. See Lowe, "Army Lifts Quota Ban" and Hine, *Black Women in White*, 181.

128. Commenting on the "Draft Nurse Bill," a number of nurses focused on the discriminatory nature of the bill in singling out women nurses. "Notes on the Draft Nurse Bill," *Trained Nurse and Hospital Review*, April 1945, 258.

129. "Nurses' Draft," *Trained Nurse and Hospital Review*, February 1945, 114.

130. According to the 1940 U.S. Census and the American Nurses' Association, there were just over eight thousand male nurses in the United States and just over seven thousand African American nurses in the United States. These numbers included those practicing and students. By January 1943 about three hundred men nurses self-reported serving in one branch of the armed forces. American Nurses' Association, *Facts about Nursing* (1943), 12; and American Nurses' Association, *Facts about Nursing* (1946), 18.

131. The national poll focused on the nursing care received from women; no mention was made to the use or commissioning of male nurses in the Army Nurse Corps. "Army Opposes Anti-Bias Clause in Nurse Draft," *Chicago Defender*, February 24, 1945, 1.

132. Janet Geister, "Plain Talk," *Trained Nurse and Hospital Review*, March 1945, 206.

Chapter 3. Nurse or Soldier?

1. As early as a year before the United States entered World War II, the army organized how occupations would be classified under the draft. Male nurses were classified as medical technicians and held a Red Cross identification card with the serial number 123. Interestingly, male nurses, like female nurses, were registered with the Red Cross, and it was the Red Cross that maintained this registry, not the War Department. Albert G. Love, Col., to Lt. Col. Herbert Holdridge, October 2, 1940, "Occupational Specialists to Be Assigned to the Medical Department," Army Nurse Corps Archives, Office of the Surgeon General [hereinafter ANCA, OSG], Falls Church, Va., box 110.

2. Mobilization propaganda focused mainly on white, middle-class women. Working-class and minority women had long been in the workforce, but war mobilization did provide some of them expanded access to better-paying jobs. Maureen Honey, *Creating Rosie the Riveter: Class, Gender, and Propaganda during WWII* (Amherst: University of Massachusetts Press, 1984); and Leila Rupp, *Mobilizing Women for War: German and American Propaganda, 1939–1945* (Princeton, N.J.: Princeton University Press, 1978).

3. Ruth Milkman, *Gender at Work: The Dynamics of Job Segregation by Sex During World War II* (Urbana: University of Illinois Press, 1987); and Alice Kessler-Harris, *Out to Work: A History of Wage-Earning Women in the United States* (1982; Oxford: Oxford University Press, 2003).

4. Portions of this chapter are also found in "The hands that might save them: Gender, race, and the politics of nursing during World War II," *Gender and History* (August 2012): 456–74. Evelyn Brooks Higginbotham, "African American Women's History and the Metalanguage of Race," *Signs* 17, no. 2 (Winter 1992): 251–74.

5. Very little information exists about the racial nature of the four schools that trained only men, but from all indications they did not accept black male nurses. See Appendix B herewith; American Nurses' Association, *Facts about Nursing* (Kansas City, Mo.: American Nurses' Association, 1950), 50; Christine L. Williams, *Gender Differences at Work: Women and Men in Nontraditional Occupations* (Berkeley: University of California Press, 1989), 91.

6. See Appendix C; only four states reported having more than ten black male nurses or students; twenty-one states reported no black male nurses or students. American Nurses' Association, *Facts about Nursing*, 18; and Estelle Massey Osborne, "Status and Contribution of the Negro Nurse," *Journal of Negro Education* 18, no. 3 (1949): 367.

7. Williams, *Gender Differences at Work*, 156; and D'Antonio, *American Nursing*, 160–63.

8. Assistant Secretary NAACP to Miss Gertrude Delahunt, April 11, 1940, Records, NAACP, part 15, series B, reel 9, frames 159–60.

9. Adia Harbey Wingfield, "Racializing the Glass Escalator: Reconsidering Men's Experiences with Women's Work," *Gender and Society* 23, no. 1 (February 2009): 5–26.

10. D'Antonio, *American Nursing*, 160–62.

11. The first organization dedicated to nursing education was the American Society of Superintendents of Training Schools for Nurses, founded in 1893; in 1912, they were renamed the National League for Nursing Education. This was one of three national nursing organizations that dominated the profession in the first half of the twentieth century. The other two organizations were the American Nurses' Association and the National Organization for Public Health Nursing, founded in 1912. ANA membership requirements originally focused on alumnae associations, not individual nurses. When the group changed its name in 1910, they became open to individual membership, but only by those who belonged to alumnae associations. Reverby, *Ordered to Care*, 123–24.

12. No direct discussion about male nurses appears to have taken place regarding the ANA's bylaws; however, the qualifications for membership limited the inclusion of male nurses.

13. "Amendments to the By-Laws," *American Journal of Nursing* 30, no. 4 (April 1930): 508.

14. According to Bruce Mericle, even at the same nursing school, women and men received different instruction at the end of the nineteenth century. This meant the women were kept from receiving instruction in urology in the same way men were kept from obstetrics. However, by all accounts, because women received more general nurse training, they probably had more contact with patients in these areas than male nurses did with obstetrics. The Mills School of Nursing for Men did not offer a course in obstetrics until 1957. Mericle, "Male as Psychiatric Nurse," 30–31; and O'Lynn and Tranbarger, *Men in Nursing*, 44–46.

15. Kenneth T. Crummer, "A School of Nursing for Men," *American Journal of Nursing* 24, no. 6 (March 1924): 459.

16. M.H.R., "Male Nurses in our Profession," *American Journal of Nursing* 24, no. 10 (July 1924): 837.

17. "Proceedings from the Nineteenth Annual Convention of the American Nurses' Association," *American Journal of Nursing* 16, no. 9 (June 1916): 787–957; and American Nurses' Association, "Basic Historical Review," American Nurses' Association, available at http://nursingworld.org/FunctionalMenuCategories/AboutANA/History/BasicHistoricalReview.pdf (accessed on August 20, 2014); and O'Lynn and Tranbarger, *Men in Nursing*, 28–29.

18. As late as 1940, the ANA continued to deliberate their membership requirements concerning African American nurses. At that time, the only black nurse members who did not belong to their state associations were alumnae members of the Freedman's Hospital in Washington, D.C., because the association was a member of the ANA before the 1916 bylaw changes. To compensate for this problem, the National League of Nursing Education changed its membership laws in 1940 to accept black nurses who belonged to the National Association of Colored Graduate Nurses. "The Philadelphia Biennial," *American Journal of Nursing* 40, no. 6 (June 1940): 677 and 684.

19. For most of its existence, the *American Journal of Nursing* was the organ for the American Nurses' Association, the National League of Nursing Education, and the majority of state nursing associations.

20. Emphasis added. M.H.R., "Male Nurses," 837.

21. Lavinia L. Dock, "Equal Rights," *American Journal of Nursing* 24, no. 10 (July 1924): 843.

22. Kenneth T. Crummer, "Male Nurses: A Survey of the Present-Day Situation of Graduate Male Nurses," *American Journal of Nursing* 28, no. 5 (May 1928): 467–69.

23. M.H.R.'s letter to the editor noted that an amendment was submitted to the national association to substitute genitourinary training for men for obstetrical and

children's training for women as a requirement for membership. This amendment failed to bring "graduate male nurses into active membership." It would be another six years before male nurses would achieve national professional recognition from the ANA. M.H.R., "Male Nurses," 837.

24. Crummer suggested that the reason for this expansion was a combination of improvements in nurse education, younger nurse students than in previous years, and different attitudes among male nurses and about male nurse occupation opportunities. Crummer, "Male Nurses," 467.

25. "Amendments to the By-Laws," 508.

26. "The Census Looks at Nurses," *American Journal of Nursing* 40, no. 2 (February 1940): 136.

27. Unlike the National Association of Colored Graduate Nurses, who by the mid-1930s had revamped their organization to launch a full-scale campaign to fight black nurse discrimination, male nurses in the United States lacked a national "male nurse" body to proceed with such an undertaking and were instead left with few prominent and outspoken male nurses to call attention to the cause. Furthermore, until the late 1930s, no state association had a separate committee or section dedicated to male nurses; branches of the New York State Nurse Associations began organizing "men nurse sections" in the late 1930s.

28. Crummer, "Male Nurses," 468.

29. J. Frederick Painton, "The Outlook in Male Nursing," *American Journal of Nursing* 37, no. 3 (March 1937): 281.

30. Frances W. Witte, "Opportunities in Graduate Education for Men Nurses," *American Journal of Nursing* 34, no. 2 (February 1934): 135; and Frederick W. Jones, "Vocational Opportunities for Men Nurses," *American Journal of Nursing* 34, no. 2 (February 1934): 131–33.

31. Crummer, "School of Nursing," 457.

32. Witte, "Opportunities," 135.

33. Crummer, "School of Nursing," 457–58; and LeRoy Craig, "Opportunities for Male Nurses," *American Journal of Nursing* 40, no. 6 (June 1940): 666–70.

34. The NLNE worked directly with the ANA (and vice versa) to promote and direct the field of professional nursing in the United States.

35. A state association with a high number of men nurses asked the board of directors for the ANA to solicit the Red Cross to change its policies excluding men.

36. The Red Cross Nursing Service was established in 1909 with the help of Jane Delano, the superintendent of the Army Nurse Corps. Its purpose was to develop a reserve for the Army Nurse Corps and to augment local nursing services in times of emergency or disaster. The Red Cross Nursing Service also provided a variety of basic aid classes to women in local communities. Virginia Dunbar and Gertrude S. Banfield, "Red Cross Nursing Service Contemplates Changes in Enrolment Plan," *American Journal of Nursing* 46, no. 2 (February 1946): 82; and Jane A. Delano, "Red Cross Work," *American Journal of Nursing* 9, no. 8 (May 1909): 582–83.

37. "No Male Red Cross Nurses," *American Journal of Nursing* 35, no. 4 (April 1935): 388.

38. Some men felt insulted by the nursing service's concession to male nurses. In light of the nursing service's limited use of male nurses, they refused to register with the Red Cross, pointing out that they had more control over their professional lives and more opportunity in the private sector if they did not register. "Red Cross Enrolls Men Nurses as Technologists," *American Journal of Nursing* 40, no. 4 (April 1940): 453; Craig, "Opportunities for Male Nurses," 670; and "Male Nurses and the Armed Forces," *American Journal of Nursing* 43, no. 12 (December 1943): 1066–69.

39. Crummer, "School of Nursing," 459.

40. "What Can We Do Now?" *American Journal of Nursing* 40, no. 7 (July 1940): 795; see also "Red Cross Nursing and the Army," *American Journal of Nursing* 40, no. 7 (July 1940): 791–94.

41. "Nursing Council on National Defense," *American Journal of Nursing* 40, no. 9 (September 1940): 1013.

42. Several state nursing associations followed suit and formed their own Men Nurse Sections in the six months following the biennial convention. This included Massachusetts, Pennsylvania, and Tennessee, to name a few. "The Philadelphia Biennial," *American Journal of Nursing* 40, no. 6 (June 1940): 678; and "News about Nursing," *American Journal of Nursing* 40, no. 12 (December 1940): 1404–38.

43. "Nursing in Democracy," *American Journal of Nursing* 40, no. 6 (June 1940): 671–72; and O'Lynn and Tranbarger, *Men in Nursing*, 29.

44. Patrick Clerkin from Central Islip State Hospital in New York was elected as the temporary first chair of the section; by 1942, LeRoy Craig had become the chair of the Men Nurses' Section. See Appendix B. In the 1940 ANA census, the organization noted that there were roughly eight thousand male nurses in the United States. Of these, two thousand were active graduate and three thousand were student male nurses available for military service. "The Philadelphia Biennial," *AJN*, 678.

45. While Craig noted that qualified male nurses could join the military as noncommissioned officers, the reality proved different. In most cases, male nurses entered the service as privates or ensigns and only later, after months of service, moved to a higher rank. Craig, "Opportunities for Male Nurses," 70.

46. Medical technicians in the army, also known as medics, were privates in the Medical Department. Their rank placed them in the position under female nurses in the ANC. Both doctors and nurses supervised them. After a number of months of service and provided a vacancy existed, medics could eventually obtain the rank of technical sergeant. Given that female nurses entered the military as officers, male nurses did not view this proposal as a welcome opportunity. "Male Nurses," 1066–69.

47. According to a memo written by Hon. Charles B. Smith, dated April 13, 1918, a group of seven male nurses located at Base Hospital 25 in France petitioned the Army Medical Corps to be classified as nurses instead of orderlies. This request was denied but reveals that World War II was not the first time male nurses attempted

to integrate the ANC; it was during World War II that their campaign was considerably larger, more organized, and much more public. "Proud to Serve: The Evolution of Male Army Nurse Corps Officers," available at http://history.amedd.army.mil/ancwebsite/articles/malenurses.html (accessed August 20, 2014).

48. Sandy F. Mannino to Franklin D. Roosevelt, June 13, 1940, ANCA, OSG, box 110.

49. Nathaniel H. Wooding to Col. Albert G. Love, July 5, 1940, ANCA, OSG, box 110.

50. Between June and December 1940, the Office of the Surgeon General received or forwarded a number of letters concerning the position of male nurses within the army. About a dozen of these were included as basic information on the topic, beginning with a letter from Joseph O'Connell to President Roosevelt, December 18, 1940, ANCA, OSG, box 110.

51. Edward F. Perreault to Franklin D. Roosevelt, October 10, 1940, ANCA, OSG, box 110.

52. Once the United States entered the war, age limits were expanded to require men between ages eighteen and forty-five to register with their local draft board. Those men of age excluded from the draft included conscientious objectors and men labeled as "necessary" to the work they were already doing in the civilian or government service sector. Interestingly enough, according to historian Timothy Stewart-Winter a large number of conscientious objectors were classified as I-A-O. This meant that they objected only to combatant service and "typically served as medics . . . in the military." My focus here is on graduate trained nurses, however, and for this reason will not discuss the I-A-O medic as part of the conversation. Timothy Stewart-Winter, "Not a Soldier, Not a Slacker: Conscientious Objectors and Male Citizenship in the United States during the Second World War," *Gender and History* 19, no. 3 (November 2007): 519–42.

53. Col. Albert G. Love to Lt. Col. Herbert Holdridge, October 2, 1940, ANCA, OSG, box 110; "Male Nurses and the Armed Services," 1066; and "Male Nurse," ANCA, OSG, box 110.

54. Mitchell Blake to Sen. Henry C. Lodge, December 7, 1940, ANCA, OSG, box 110.

55. "Red Cross Nursing Service Enrollments," *American Journal of Nursing* 41, no. 12 (December 1941): 1452.

56. LeRoy Craig to Col. Albert G. Love, July 6, 1940, ANCA, OSG, box 110.

57. American Nurses' Association, "Re Status of Male Nurses in the Army and Navy," January 13, 1942, from document "Resume of Actions Taken by American Nurses' Association with Regard to Securing Recognition of Male Nurses Serving in the Armed Forces," January 9, 1943, ANCA, OSG, box 110.

58. Love rarely defined what he meant by "administrative problems" but did allude to it in a memo he typed on behalf of the surgeon general. Here, he suggests that managing the nurse corps, including basic efforts like housing, would be impossible with the inclusion of male nurses. Furthermore, unlike female nurses who were appointed to one job, male service members were expected to be flexible and able to

perform whatever duties were needed of them to support the mission of the army. Memo located with Joseph P. D. O'Connell to President Roosevelt, December 18, 1940, ANCA, OSG, box 110; Henry L. Stimson to Robert R. Reynolds, April 5, 1944, *Records of the War Department*, RG 165, NARA, box 181.

59. H. Richard Musser, "Nurse or Soldier," *American Journal of Nursing* 41, no. 12 (December 1941): 1449.

60. American Nurses' Association, "Service of Male Nurses during War," 1942, ANCA, OSG, box 110, pp. 1–3.

61. American Nurses' Association, "Service of Male Nurses," 11.

62. Nathaniel H. Wooding to Col. Albert G. Love, September 7, 1940; and Col. Albert G. Love to Nathaniel H. Wooding, October 1, 1940, ANCA, OSG, box 110. Nathaniel H. Wooding, "Nursing Is an Essential Occupation," *American Journal of Nursing* 41, no. 7 (July 1941): 838.

63. The National Nursing Council for War Service was established in 1940 as the Nursing Council for National Defense and changed its name in 1942. The group helped coordinate nursing resources with representatives from nursing organizations, nursing schools, and the U.S. military, providing guidance and support on nursing during World War II.

64. Honey, *Creating Rosie the Riveter*; and Rupp, *Mobilizing Women for War*.

65. American Nurses' Association, "Service of Male Nurses," 1–3.

66. American Nurses' Association, "Resume of Actions," 1–4; and John K. Welch to Col. Florence A. Blanchfield, July 24, 1943, ANCA, OSG, box 110.

67. R. A. Chiniok to Lt. Cuppy, December 6, 1943, France P. Bolton Papers, Western Reserve Historical Society, Cleveland, Ohio, folder 140 [hereinafter WRHS].

68. "Male Nurses," [1943?], ANCA, OSG, box 110; Williams, *Gender Differences at Work*, 40–42.

69. J. Beatrice Bowman, "The Pharmacist's Mates' School," *American Journal of Nursing* 27, no. 7 (July 1927): 523–27; and Miriam M. Bryan to Frances P. Bolton, February 19, 1945, Frances P. Bolton Papers, WRHS, folder 140.

70. "Relative rank" allowed a woman in this still-auxiliary group to receive pay commensurate with that of commissioned officers of the same rank, but not all other rights and privileges. Col. Florence A. Blanchfield to John K. Welch, August 6, 1943, ANCA, OSG, box 110.

71. Sarnecky, *History*, 50–51 and 56–57.

72. Ibid., 146–47.

73. Blanchfield to Welch, August 6, 1943; and "Male Nurses," 1943, ANCA, OSG, box 110.

74. Leslie, Capt. C. J. to John Livingstone, April 1, 1943, "Ref. to Men Joining the ANC," ANCA, OSG, box 110.

75. See Appendix A; see also chapter 2.

76. National Association for Colored Graduate Nurses and the National Nursing Council for War Service, February 21, 1945, *Facts about Negro Nurses and the War* (New York: NACGN and NNCWS Headquarters, 1945) OSG, ANCA, box 108.

77. Nursing estimates suggested that there were about eight thousand male nurses practicing during the war; however, only about two thousand of them were qualified for military service. Further, the 320 male nurses serving with the armed forces in 1943 worked in a variety of areas, not all of which were the Medical Department. "Male Nurses and the Armed Services," 1067.

78. In an interesting reversal of recognition of graduate male nurses entering the military, an ex-pharmacist's mate, who served in the navy for eight years, introduced a bill would allow men who served four or more years in the Army and Navy Medical Departments recognition as "registered male nurses" once they left the military. The question of professional recognition was not limited to males who already had graduate nursing degrees, however, given the limited training pharmacist's mates and medical technicians received, the prospect that this would occur was very limited. American Nurses' Association, "Service of Male Nurses," 9; Herbert B. Schiek to Dr. Geo. Baehr, January 30, 1943, ANCA, OSG, box 110.

79. Sarnecky, *History*, 268–69.

80. Frances P. Bolton to Joseph R. Guerra, May 17, 1944, and Frances P. Bolton to 1st Sergeant Donald E. Zboray, January 18, 1945, Frances P. Bolton Papers, WRHS, folder 140.

81. H.R. 4760 was superseded by H.R. 68 and H.R. 483. Victor Neu to Congressman Hadwen C. Fuller, January 15, 1945, Frances P. Bolton Papers, WRHS, folder 140.

82. The president signed H.R. 4445 on June 22, 1944, giving female nurse officers temporary commissions in the army. Sarnecky, *History*, 269.

83. Norman T. Kirk to Frances P. Bolton, December 27, 1944, Frances P. Bolton Papers, WRHS, folder 141.

84. Ibid.

85. It is almost impossible to gain a true measure of the nursing shortage during World War II. Recruitment campaigns since before the war called female nurses to join the ranks of the understaffed Nurse Corps. The request became more vocal beginning in 1943, and most citizens understood that as the fighting increased, the need for nurses increased exponentially. Julia Flikke, "The Army Calls All Eligible Nurses," *American Journal of Nursing* 43, no. 1 (January 1943): 25; and Maj. Edna B. Groppe, "Statements Made at the Public Hearing before the House Military Affairs Committee on February 14, 1945," *American Journal of Nursing* 45, no. 3 (March 1945): 175.

86. "Seek 8,500 More Nurses," *New York Times*, July 18, 1944; Mabel K. Staupers, "Negro Nurses Would Serve," *New York Times*, December 15, 1944; "Suggests Negro Nurses," *New York Times*, January 12, 1945; "Would Use Negro Nurses," *New York Times*, January 21, 1945; "Army Lifts Ban on Negro Nurses," *PM*, July 12, 1944; Congress, House, *Message from the President of the United States*, 79th Congress, 1st session, January 6, 1945, document 1, p. 7; and Maj. Gen. Norman Kirk as quoted in "Nurses Face Draft as Casualties Rise," *Stars and Stripes*, Sunday, January 7, 1945, ANCA, OSG, box 79.

87. Groppe, "Statements," 175.

88. Robert Cincotta to Frances P. Bolton, January 24, 1945, Frances P. Bolton Papers, WRHS, folder 140.

89. John W. Martyn (OSG) to Hon. J. Hardin Peterson, January 17, 1945, ANCA, OSG, box 110.

90. W. J. C. Agnew to Frances P. Bolton, February 13, 1945, Frances P. Bolton Papers, WRHS, folder 140.

91. Alfred Reetz to Frances P. Bolton, January 28, 1945, Frances P. Bolton Papers, WRHS, folder 140; Katherine J. Densford, "Statement Made by Katherine J. Densford before the Senate Military Affairs Committee, March 23, 1945," *American Journal of Nursing* 45 (May 1945): 384; and Edith Nourse Rogers Papers, SL-RI, box 1, folder 15.

92. Pvt. James L. Ortasic to Frances P. Bolton, January 19, 1945, Frances P. Bolton Papers, WRHS, folder 140.

93. Minnie Goodnow to Frances P. Bolton, December 6, 1944, Frances P. Bolton Papers, WRHS, folder 140.

94. Frances P. Bolton to Dan Wacks, February 17, 1945, Frances P. Bolton Papers, WRHS, folder 140.

95. The January 20, 1945, declaration by the surgeon general is a little misleading, as it pertained to African American nurses. Officially, the army lifted the quotas or "Jim Crow" ban of black nurses in early July 1944, but getting African American nurses appointed was still difficult; disheartened by continued racist treatment, many black nurses stopped trying to join the ANC. The January 20 declaration took the July 1944 end to quotas a step further, ensuring that all qualified female nurses would be accepted. Lowe, "Army Lifts Quota Ban"; and Hine, *Black Women in White*, 181.

96. The poll focused on the nursing care provided by women, but no mention was made to the use or commissioning of male nurses in the Army Nurse Corps. "Army Opposes Anti-Bias Clause in Nurse Draft," *Chicago Defender*, February 24, 1945, 1.

97. *Congressional Record*, March 5, 1945, 1729; and Beatrice Kalisch and Philip Kalisch, "The Women's Draft," *Nursing Research* 22, no. 5 (September–October 1973): 408.

98. Edith M. Beattie, "Nurse Draft Legislation and the ANA—A Summary," *American Journal of Nursing* 45, no. 7 (July 1945): 547.

99. "Nurse Draft: Pro/Con," *Trained Nurse and Hospital Review* (February 1945): 114–15.

100. Hine, *Black Women in White*, 182–83; Sarnecky, *History*, 271; Densford, "Statement"; and Beattie, "Nurse Draft Legislation," 547–48.

101. Frances P. Bolton to Dan Wacks, February 17, 1945, Frances P. Bolton Papers, WRHS, folder 140.

Chapter 4. An American Challenge

1. Margaret Culkin Banning, "Women in a Defense Decade," *American Journal of Nursing* 51, no. 12 (December 1951): 748–49.

2. The use of anticommunism to both hinder and help social justice activities is not new in the postwar period. It has been employed, according to historians Peter J. Kuznick and James Gilbert, as early as the 1880s against labor and later by New

Dealers. Kuznick and Gilbert, eds., *Rethinking Cold War Culture* (Washington: Smithsonian Institution Press, 2001), 7–9.

3. As we will see later in the chapter, both female and male nurses used gendered understandings of work as a strategy to further their own purposes. Kessler-Harris, *In Pursuit of Equity*, 204.

4. In 1944 President Roosevelt signed H.R. 4445. This gave army nurses temporary commission in the regular army for the duration of the war and six months following the end of hostilities. The 1947 act made female nurses and the ANC permanent members of the regular army.

5. Earl Lomon Koos, "What Society Demands of the Nurse," *American Journal of Nursing* 47, no. 5 (May 1947): 306.

6. Florence A. Blanchfield, "New Status in Military Nursing: Peacetime Opportunities in the Army Nurse Corps," *American Journal of Nursing* 47, no. 9 (September 1947): 604.

7. Margaret Chase Smith actually introduced the 1947 bill, but Frances Bolton had suggested the striking of "female" from the law. This was in line with her goal of opening the armed forces nurses corps and expanding the nursing profession to women and men, all races, creeds, and ethnicities. Sarnecky, *History*, 219–92.

8. Together, the Army-Navy Nurse Act of 1947 and the Women's Armed Services Integration Act of 1948 provided women a permanent place in the armed forces of the United States. Linda Witt, Judith Bellafaire, Britts Granrud, and Mary Jo Binker, *"A Defense Weapon Known to Be of Value": Servicewomen of the Korean Conflict Era* (Hanover, N.H.: University Press of New England, 2005), 31–33.

9. Frances P. Bolton, "FPB Comments: Nursing-Health," Frances P. Bolton Papers, WRHS, folder 55, pp. 201–2; and "Nurses' Non-Bias Clause Defeated," *Chicago Defender*, March 22, 1947.

10. Manfred Berg, "Black Civil Rights and Liberal Anticommunism: The NAACP in the Early Cold War," *Journal of American History* 94, no. 1 (June 2007): 75–96.

11. Franklin D. Roosevelt's "Four Freedoms" speech to Congress in January 1941 provided civil rights activists with a presidential mandate to base their argument for equal rights, including social and economic security and civil liberties. Available at http://www.fdrlibrary.marist.edu/pdfs/ffreadingcopy.pdf (accessed on August 10, 2014); Penny Von Eschen, *Satchmo Blows up the World: Jazz Ambassadors Play the Cold War* (Cambridge, Mass.: Harvard University Press, 2004).

12. After a long legal battle by the NAACP, the Supreme Court declared white primaries in Texas unconstitutional in *Smith v. Allwright* in 1944. The case had widespread implications. It helped double the number of blacks in southern states registered to vote by 1950 and bolstered membership in the NAACP.

13. Although the military remained segregated throughout World War II, African Americans did earn recognition for their service to the country. Ulysses Lee, *The Employment of Negro Troops* (Washington, D.C.: Center for Military History, 1994); Martha Putney, *When the Nation Was in Need: Blacks in the Women's Army Corps during WWII* (Metuchen, N.J.: Scarecrow, 1992); and Lawrence P. Scott, *Double V:*

The Civil Rights Struggle of the Tuskegee Airman (East Lansing: Michigan State University Press, 1994).

14. For more information on the Detroit Riot, see Thomas J. Sugrue, *Origins of the Urban Crisis: Race and Inequality in Postwar Detroit* (Princeton, N.J: Princeton University Press, 2005), chapter 2.

15. One of the more infamous cases of racial violence occurred with the ambush and murder of Roger Malcolm and George Dorsey and their wives. Malcolm and Dorsey were both returning veterans who, to the Ku Klux Klan, represented African Americans "getting out of their place." Steven F. Lawson, ed., *To Secure These Rights* (New York: Bedford/St. Martin, 2004), 8; Mary L. Dudziak, *Cold War Civil Rights*, 18–19.

16. Gunnar Mrydal's 1944 release of *An American Dilemma* detailed the damage that racism had done and would do to the future of the United States. It was published during the period when the wartime alliance between the Soviet Union and United States began to break down. The United States' history of discrimination against its racial minorities became important in the postwar struggle to gain the hearts and favor of recent independent nations and in the Third World. Civil rights activists attempted to use this situation as a strategy to push their domestic civil rights agenda, with varying degrees of success.

17. The National Emergency Committee against Mob Violence consisted of the "NAACP and at least forty other civil rights, labor, religious, and veterans' groups." Lawson, *To Secure These Rights*, 9.

18. The PCCR often used the terms civil liberties and civil rights interchangeably, drawing attention in their recommendation to not only those rights covered by the Thirteenth, Fourteenth, and Fifteenth Amendments but also those liberties covered by the Bill of Rights. Ibid., 12–24.

19. Ibid., iv.

20. "NACGN Joins in Asking Civil Rights Action by Congress," *National News Bulletin* 2, no. 3 (September 1948) in the Records of the NACGN, reel 1.

21. The committee's recommendations were farreaching. They touched on everything from housing to education, the role of the Justice Department, and future civil rights legislation. Many of the recommendations would be difficult to achieve in the ensuing years, and Truman understood that perhaps little to nothing would come from the report. However, the report's emphasis on the responsibility of the federal government to protect the civil rights of all its citizens had lasting effects. Ultimately, the report served as a "blueprint" for fighting Jim Crow for both the Federal Government and civil rights activists. Lawson, *To Secure These Rights*, 28–31 and 167–85.

22. The eruption of Cold War tensions between 1946 and 1948 drove Truman to recognize the possibility of another draft to prepare the military for war. Dudziak, *Cold War Civil Rights*, 84.

23. Harry S. Truman, "Special Message to Congress," February 2, 1948, digital collection, Truman Presidential Library, available at http://trumanlibrary.org/publicpapers/index.php?pid=1380 (accessed August 20, 2014).

24. Christine Knauer, *Let Us Fight as Free Men: Black Soldiers and Civil Rights* (Philadelphia: University of Pennsylvania Press, 2014), 112–13.

25. "President Truman wipes out segregation in Armed Forces," *Chicago Defender*, July 31, 1948, and Lem Graves, "Army Bias Probe Starts: It Can End Segregation—Will It?" *Pittsburgh Courier*, January 15, 1949.

26. John Lewis Gaddis, *The Cold War: A New History* (New York: Penguin, 2005), 25–47.

27. "Hints FBI Will Probe Youths Who Boycott Segregated Conscription," *Chicago Defender*, July 31, 1948, 4.

28. Sarnecky, *History*, 316.

29. Registered nurse Earl McDowell praises Bolton's bill to "eliminate sex discrimination in the Armed Forces." "FBP Comments: Nursing-Health," Frances P. Bolton Papers, WRHS, folder 61, pp. 248, 258, and 261; Earl McDowell to Frances P. Bolton, 1950, Frances P. Bolton Papers, WRHS, folder 140; "Sex Discrimination," *RN* 13 (September 1950): 60; and "Male, Negro Nurses Urged in Emergency," *New York Times*, March 14, 1951, 8.

30. MacLean, *Freedom Is Not Enough*, 38.

31. The purpose of the intergroup program was twofold. First, it formed as a group to deal with internal relations, which included dealing with problems surrounding economic security, job placement, and counseling. Second, in an external capacity the group acted as a liaison with other community groups that were concerned with discrimination. "Intergroup Relations," *American Journal of Nursing* 55, no. 9 (September 1955): 1061.

32. The Intergroup Relations Committee most often discussed discrimination as it pertained to race; however, as the 1956 description of its policies pointed out, the group fought discrimination against any "race, creed, color or sex." Therefore, a discussion of minority nurses most often included not only black nurses but also male nurses. "ANA Policies on Intergroup Relations," *American Journal of Nursing* 56, no. 2 (February 1956): 167.

33. Passed in 1946, the Hill-Burton Act provided federal and state money for the expansion of hospitals and medical care; adequate nursing staff was important to this expansion. D'Antonio, *American Nursing*, 167–68.

34. Nurse Illustration, *National News Bulletin* 4, no. 2 (December 1950), Records of the NACGN, reel 1.

35. In general, the race of male nurses was not noted on tables listing the number of male nurses admitted to and graduated from nursing schools. Further, the statistics on African American nurses admitted and graduated did not list the sex of the nurses. One rare document, however, does indicate that of the "774 men enrolled in nursing schools in 1949, 16 were negroes." "Nursing Schools at the Mid-Century National Committee for Improvement of Nursing Services, New York 1950," ANCA, OSG, box 110a; and American Nurses' Association, *Facts about Nursing*, 1950, 38; and American Nurses' Association, "House of Delegates Proceedings," May 1950, American Nurses' Association Collection, HGARC; see also Appendix D herewith.

36. By 1956, the ANA's board of directors formally acknowledged their opinion that Congress had a responsibility to act on civil rights legislation. American Nurses' Association, "Committee on Legislation," 41st Convention, House of Delegates Section Reports, 1956–1958, American Nurses' Association Collection, HGARC, 126.

37. Estelle Massey Osborne served as president of the NACGN during the mid-1930s and was instrumental, along with Mabel K. Staupers, in placing the black nurse cause on a national civil rights agenda. Hine, *Black Women in White*, 183.

38. Until he resigned in protest, Hastie served as the civilian liaison for race relations to the Secretary of War on civil rights during World War II. He is considered a pioneer in the civil rights movement. Judge William Hastie, "Speech from the Testimonial Dinner of the NACGN," Mabel K. Staupers Papers, MSRC, Washington, D.C., box 96-2, folder 35.

39. Langston Hughes, "Where Service is Needed," in *A Salute to Democracy at Mid-Century*, January 26, 1951, NACGN Records, 1908–1951, reel 2.

40. Although "minority" was and is commonly used to refer to a racial "other," in the case of nursing it was used to describe any group of nurses not of the majority, white or female. Some were African American female nurses—those who joined before 1916 or who lived in a state that allowed them membership in their State Nursing Association. It was not until 1948 that the bylaws were changed to allow nurses who did not hold membership in their state associations to join the national body.

41. The number of training schools open to African Americans and men nurses nearly tripled between 1940 and 1950, from 76 to 207 and from 68 to 183, respectively. American Nurses' Association, *Facts about Nursing*, 1950, 46–47.

42. "Women and War," *RN* 13 (October 1950): 57.

43. The American Nurses' Association noted in a summer issue of its journal that steps were taken to "initiate legislation granting military rank to male nurses." In December 1949, Col. Mary G. Phillips, chief of the ANC, solicited her chief officers about the possible addition of men in the corps. "Congress Considers Nursing," *American Journal of Nursing* 49, no. 7 (July 1949): 429.

44. Female officers' responses to Colonel Phillips's notification mentioned her December 30, 1949, letter to them. "Gender-Male Nurses," ANCA, OSG, box 110a.

45. Col. Phillips's request yielded several dozen letters from female nurse officers. ANCA, OSG, boxes 110 and 110a.

46. Lt. Col. Katharine V. Jolliffe to Col. Mary G. Phillips, January 9, 1950, ANCA, OSG, box 110a.

47. "Gendered imagination" is the processes by which social policies and social relationships are constructed and sustained. They are so much a part of social society that they are thought of as "normal," with little acknowledgment to how they are historically constructed or retooled to support particular divisions between the sexes. Kessler-Harris, *In Pursuit of Equity*, 18 and 204.

48. "Acceptance of Male Nurses in Army Nurse Corps," January 1950, ANCA, OSG, box 110a.

49. "War Neuroses Subcommittee Minutes," May 1, 1941, NARA, RG 215; "Acceptance of Male Nurses in Army Nurse Corps," January 1950; and Lt. Col. Ruby F. Bryant to Col. Mary G. Phillips, January 6, 1950, ANCA, OSG, box 110a.

50. Lt. Col. Bryant to Col. Phillips, January 6, 1950.

51. Ibid.; Lt. Col. Daisy McCommons to Col. Mary G. Phillips, January 5, 1950; and Lt. Col. Ida W. Danielson to Col. Mary G. Phillips, January 18, 1950, all located at ANCA, OSG, box 110a.

52. See Appendix D herewith. According to the American Nurses' Association's records, in 1950 there were ten thousand men nurses registered in the United States, or about 6 percent of the total civilian population. "Acceptance of Male Nurses."

53. According to retired Brigadier General Lillian Dunlap, the military believed men were best suited to orthopedics, genitourinary wards, and psychiatry wards. These were indeed the wards where men initially worked. She also noted that some officials and doctors were uncomfortable with male nurses on wards where they cared for women or children because of a fear of improprieties. Lillian Dunlap, *33 Years of Army Nursing: An Interview with Brigadier General Lillian Dunlap.* Conducted by Cynthia A. Gurney (U.S. Army Nurse Corps: Washington, D.C., 2001), 105–6.

54. Maj. Francis C. Gunn to Col. Mary G. Phillips, January 16, 1950, ANCA, OSG, box 110a.

55. It was not until 1964 that married women could gain initial appointment in the ANC and have dependents under the age of fifteen. Sarnecky, *History*, 272; and Carolyn M. Feller and Constance Moore, *Highlights in the History of the Army Nurse Corps* (Washington, D.C.: U.S. Army Center of Military History, 1995), 18 and 38.

56. Maj. Naomi J. Jensen to Col. Mary G. Phillips, January 10, 1950; and Lt. Col. Daisy McCommons to Col. Mary G. Phillips, January 18, 1950, ANCA, OSG, box 110a.

57. Ruby F. Bryant to Col. H. W. Glattly, July 22, 1952, "Study of Utilizing Graduate Professional Male Nurses within the Army," ANCA, OSG, box 110.

58. Katherine E. Baltz, December 28, 1949, "Policies and Laws Governing Male Nurses," ANCA, OSG, box 110a.

59. Fifteen percent of women chose teaching, making it the second on the list of professions for women. George H. Gallup, *Gallup Poll—Public Opinion, 1949–1958* vol. 2 (New York: Random House, 1972), 892.

60. Lt. Col. Rosalie D. Colhoun to Col. Mary G. Phillips, January 3, 1950, ANCA, OSG, box 110a.

61. Short's comments are not entirely correct as a committee of psychiatrists during the previous war indicated a preference for male nurses. "War Neuroses"; Lt. Col. Augusta L. Short to Col. Mary G. Phillips, January 16, 1950, ANCA, OSG, box 110a.

62. Maj. Mabel G. Stott to Col. Mary G. Phillips, January 23, 1950; and Lt. Col. Elsie E. Schneider to Col. Mary G. Phillips, January 26, 1950, ANCA, OSG, box 110a.

63. Celeste K. Kemler, "Our Operating Room Supervisor Is a Man," *American Journal of Nursing* 49, no. 6 (June 1949): 336.

64. Short to Phillips, January 16, 1950.

65. These fears were not unfounded: in the civilian nursing profession, the career track for many male nurses took them into administrative positions.

66. Colhoun to Phillips, January 3, 1950.

67. "Acceptance of Male Nurses."

68. Ibid.

69. Col. Mildred I. Clark, interviewed by Lt. Col. Nancy R. Adams, 1986, vol. 1, transcript, ANCA, 165–66.

70. For a detailed discussion of Frances P. Bolton's legislative attempts, see Susan Cramer Winters, "Enlightened Citizen: Frances Payne Bolton and the Nursing Profession," PhD diss., University of Virginia, 1997: 299–301; and Sarnecky, *History*, 297.

71. Representatives from the ANA among others met with the surgeon general's office and other members of the United States' military to discuss the possibility of male nurse inclusion and the provisions of the bill introduced by Congresswoman Bolton. Maj. George Armstrong to Satterlee, Warfield, and Stephens, August 15, 1950, ANCA, OSG, box 110a.

72. The other purposes of the bill included the "appointment and utilization of qualified male dietitians, physical therapists, and occupational therapists in the Women's Medical Specialist Corps on the same basis as females now appointed therein." Maj. Gen. R. W. Bliss, Surgeon General, August 31, 1950, ANCA, OSG, box 110a; Congresswoman Frances P. Bolton to Maj. Gen. R. W. Bliss, Surgeon General, August 14, 1950, ANCA, OSG, box 110a; and "A Bill," Frances P. Bolton Papers, WRHS, folder 140.

73. Earl McDowell, RN to Congresswoman Frances P. Bolton, n.d., Frances P. Bolton Papers, WRHS, folder 140; and "Sex Discrimination," *RN* (September 1950): 60.

74. "Women and War," *RN* (October 1950): 56–57.

75. Elaine Tyler May, *Homeward Bound: American Families in the Cold War Era* (New York: Basic, 1988).

76. For information on the experiences of women doctors during World War II and the Cold War, see Judith Bellafaire and Mercedes Herrera Graf, *Women Doctors in War* (College Station: Texas A&M University Press, 2009), chapters 3–5; "The Fair Sex," *RN* (September 1950): 51; and "Women and War," 57.

77. H.R. 4384 got much further than any bill on male nurses: the Senate and House passed it, but because the Committee on Armed Services failed to make the necessary modifications to the bill, it was never enacted. It was not until Public Law 408 passed in June 1952 that the appointment of qualified women physicians was authorized in the army, navy, and air force. Witt, Bellafaire, Granrud, and Binker, *"Defense Weapon,"* 132–34.

78. In an interview, Mildred I. Clark would later remember that many people viewed male nurses as having "something wrong with 'em." Mildred I. Clark, interviewed by Nancy R. Adams, p. 165; Secretary of the Army Frank Paco Jr. to Hon. Carl Vinson, October 5, 1950, ANCA, OSG, box 110a; and MBH to Bolton, October 17, 1950, Frances P. Bolton Papers, WRHS, folder 140.

79. The Fahy Committee, or the President's Committee on Equality of Treatment and Opportunity in the Armed Forces, was established as part of Executive Order 9981. It was authorized by the president to "examine rules, procedures, and practices of the armed services to determine how these might be altered or improved to bring about equality of treatment and opportunity within the military." Monroe Billington, "Freedom to Serve: The President's Committee on Equality of Treatment and Opportunity in the Armed Forces, 1949–1950," *Journal of Negro History* 51, no. 4 (October 1966): 262–74.

80. Brig. Gen. Paul I. Robinson to Mrs. Morris Earle, October 27, 1950, ANCA, OSG, box 110a.

81. H.R. 9398 is exactly the bill introduced six months later in January 1951 as H.R. 911. John A. McCart to Hon. Carl Vinson, October 18, 1950, Frances P. Bolton Papers, WRHS, folder 140; and Col. C. H. Gingles, June 18, 1951, "Use of Male Nurse by Department of Army," ANCA, OSG, box 110a.

82. Sarnecky, *History*, 297; and Mildred, interviewed by Nancy R. Adams.

83. The Joint Committee on Nursing in National Security comprised six national nursing organizations: American Nurses' Association, American Association of Industrial Nurses, Association of Collegiate Schools of Nursing, National Association of Colored Graduate Nurses, National League of Nursing Education, and National Organization for Public Health Nursing. "Mobilization of Nurses for National Security," *American Journal of Nursing* 51, no. 2 (February 1951): 78–79.

84. "Nurse Anesthetists," *RN* (November 1950): 57–58.

85. While commonly known as the Korean War, Truman never asked Congress for a declaration of war, referring to it as a "conflict" or "police action." For information on the origins of the Korean conflict and the international/Cold War implications of the hostilities, see William Stueck, *Rethinking the Korean Conflict: A New Diplomatic and Strategic History* (Princeton, N.J.: Princeton University Press, 2002).

86. Most sources place the number somewhere between five hundred and six hundred nurses, but there have been a few sources that suggest a number as high as fifteen hundred. Mildred I. Clark, "Stand By for Korea," unpublished manuscript, February 6, 1962, ANCA, OSG; Sarnecky, *History*, 295, 298, and 319; and Kalisch and Kalisch, *Advance of Nursing*, 381.

87. Sarnecky, *History*, 305.

88. John P. Wooden, "Background of Army Nurse Corps in Korea," February 12, 1951; and "Role of Army Nurse," January 29, 1951, ANCA, OSG; and "With the Army Nurse Corps in Korea," *American Journal of Nursing* 51, no. 6 (June 1951): 387.

89. The Far East Command, or FECOM, which included both Japan and Korea, became a major disputed territory between the Soviet Union and the United States during the mid-century Cold War. Wooden, "Background"; "Role of Army Nurse"; and Gaddis, *Cold War*.

90. Claude A. Barnett, "Commander Admits Army in Europe is Segregated," *Baltimore Afro-American*, March 1, 1952; "Navy Welcomes Women," *Chicago Defender*,

August 26, 1950; and "WACS in Germany Find Discrimination Disgusting," *Baltimore Afro-American*, October 13, 1951.

91. Daniel Widner, "Seoul City Sue and the Bugout Blues: Black American Narratives of the Forgotten War," in Fred Ho and Bill V. Mullen, eds., *Afro Asia: Revolutionary Political and Cultural Connections between African Americans and Asian American* (Durham, N.C.: Duke University Press, 2008), 550.

92. The military was only one of several American organizations meant to defend and promote American democracy. Von Eschen, *Satchmo*; Widner, "Seoul City Sue"; and Helen Laville and Scott Lucas, "The American Way: Edith Sampson, the NAACP, and African American Identity in the Cold War," *Diplomatic History* 20, no. 4 (Fall 1996): 565–90.

93. Dorothy B. Ferebee to Harry S. Truman, July 19, 1951, digitized collection: Truman Presidential Museum and Library.

94. T. R. Fehrenbach, *This Kind of War: A Study in Unpreparedness* (New York: Macmillan, 1963), 520, quoted in Sarnecky, *History*, 317.

95. Bailey later became the first African American nurse to reach the rank of colonel in the ANC. Bailey arrived in Germany in February 1951, accompanied by First Lieutenants Hester M. Jackson and Dorothy M. Richards. Margaret E. Bailey, *The Challenge: Autobiography of Colonel Margaret E. Bailey* (Lisle, Ill.: Tucker, 1999), 52.

96. Ibid., 52–56.

97. Sarnecky, *History*, 316.

98. Helen I. Dunne to Ida Graham Price, May 21, 1954, ANCA, OSG.

99. Robert F. Patterson to Gov. Chauncey Sparks, September 1, 1944, NARA, RG 165, box 189.

100. Dunlap, *33 Years*, 86–87.

101. Joanne Meyerowitz, "Sex, Gender, and the Cold War Language of Reform"; and Jane Sherron De Hart, "Containment at Home: Gender, Sexuality, and National Identity in Cold War America," in Kuznick and Gilbert, *Rethinking Cold War Culture*, 124–55. For a conversation on white conservative backlash, see Jason Morgan Ward, "'A War for States' Rights': The White Supremacists' Vision of Double Victory," in *Fog of War: The Second World War and the Civil Rights Movement*, edited by Kevin M. Kruse and Stephen Tuck (Cambridge: Oxford University Press, 2012), 126–44.

102. There is an underlying sense of racism in the nurse corps chief's use of the term "oriental." This was meant to differentiate the respectable and civilized "white nurse" from the "ruthless and unprincipled" other. Dorothy Brandon, "Men to Replace Nurses Up Front Urged by Korean Nurses' Leader," *New York Herald Tribune*, May 5, 1952.

103. Lt. Col. Alice M. Gritsavage, as quoted in Dorothy Brandon, "Calls Army Nurse 'Hazard to Troops,'" *Washington Post*, June 1, 1952, 17; see Brandon, "Men to Replace Nurses"; Brandon, "Nurses Prove They Can Take Korea in Stride," *New York Herald Tribune*, June 29, 1952.

104. Sixty-eight female nurses were captured by the Japanese in 1942 and held as prisoners of war for two-and-a-half years on the island of Santo Tomas. The women reported fear, degradation, unsanitary living conditions, and physical and psychological abuse at the hands of the captors. The country was reminded of this experience when questions were raised about the use of male nurses during the Korean War. Sarnecky, *History*, 186–94.

105. At least two female nurses accompanied the MASH unit to train the corpsmen to be "male nurses," one of those was Kay Phillips. She remained with the 8225th to offer support. Dorothy G. Horwitz, ed., *We Will Not Be Strangers: Korean War Letters between a M.A.S.H. Surgeon and His Wife* (Urbana: University of Illinois Press, 1997), 99 and 175.

106. Ibid., 128.

107. Ibid., 100.

108. Ibid., 131.

109. Ibid., 218–19.

110. Ibid., 229.

111. Morris A. Wolf, "Male Nurses in Services," *New York Times*, May 5, 1952.

112. Although the military resolved many of its problems with the commissioning of women physicians, they had to prove, as did female nurses, that their husbands and children were completely *dependent* on them before the military would grant the female officer dependent pay. This was not something that male officers had to prove and thus points to the fact that equality among male and female doctors did not result with the passage of Public Law 408. Instead, the same gender stereotypes remained. Men needed the dependent pay because they were the family breadwinners, while the general assumption remained that married women were not the primary means of support for the families. Witt, Bellafaire, Granrud, and Binker, *"Defense Weapon,"* 132–34.

113. Wolf, "Male Nurses in Services."

114. Italics added for emphasis. Baltz, "Policies."

115. Frances P. Bolton to Hon. Carl Vinson, September 18, 1951, Frances P. Bolton Papers, WRHS, folder 140.

116. Horwitz, *We Will Not Be Strangers*, 99, 128, 131, 175, and 218–19.

117. Clark, interviewed by Adams, 164–67.

118. Wolf, "Male Nurses in Services"; and George Chauncey, *Gay New York: Gender, Urban Culture, and the Making of the Gay Male World 1890–1940* (New York: Basic, 1994).

119. "Meeting and Workshop at the Historical Unit, Fort Detrick, Maryland," February 3, 1975, ANCA, OSG, 34–35.

120. Clark, interviewed by Adams, 165.

121. Chauncey, *Gay New York*, introduction; and John D'Emilio, "The Homosexual Menace: Sexuality in Cold War America," in *Passion and Power: Sexuality in History*, edited by Kathy Peiss and Christina Simmons (Philadelphia: Temple University Press, 1989), 226–40.

122. Bolton to Vinson, September 18, 1951.

123. In August 1953 registered nurse Duane Kirby applied for commission as a medical assistant in the Medical Service Corps but was denied because of a "lack of qualifications." Duane W. Kirby to Frances P. Bolton, August 25, 1953, Frances P. Bolton Papers, WRHS, folder 141.

124. "The Fair Sex," *RN* (September 1950): 51; "Women and War," 57; Witt, Bellafaire, Granrud, and Binker, *"Defense Weapon,"* 132–34.

125. Bolton's 1954 bill was H.R. 7898; the bill that was ultimately passed in 1955 was H.R. 2559. Frances P. Bolton, February 16, 1954, "A Bill to Authorize Male Nurses and Medical Specialists to be Appointed as Reserve Officers," Frances P. Bolton Papers, WRHS, folder 141; and LeRoy N. Craig to Anna M. Rosenberg, February 8, 1952, and March 20, 1952, Frances P. Bolton Papers, WRHS, folder 140.

126. Dien Bien Phu was the final battle between the French Union Forces and the Vietnamese Viet Minh communist revolutionary forces in 1954. It ended with the French defeat and withdrawal from its former colony.

127. *Congressional Record*, May 20, 1954, p. 6547; and Bud and Gene to Frances P. Bolton, May 19, 1954, "Suggested Statement on Male Nurses," Frances P. Bolton Papers, WRHS, folder 141.

128. President Dwight D. Eisenhower officially signed into law H.R. 2559 on August 9, 1955, which authorized reserve commissions for male nurses in the Army Nurse Corps. Sarnecky, *History*, 296–97.

129. Feller and Moore, *Highlights*, 28; and "A Salute to Male Nurses," *Washington Post*, December 30, 1955.

130. Frances P. Bolton, January 20, 1955, and Gerard Edwards to Frances P. Bolton, August 9, 1965, Frances P. Bolton Papers, WRHS, folders 141 and 142.

131. "FBP Comments: Nursing-Health," Frances P. Bolton Papers, WRHS, folders 61, 258 and 260.

Chapter 5. The Quality of a Person

1. Historian Jane Sherron De Hart discusses the struggle between social conservatives bent on domestic containment in the 1950s and 1960s and burgeoning movements aimed at "gender, sexual, and racial norms and behaviors." De Hart, "Containment at Home," 132–34.

2. Sherie Mershon and Steven Schlossman, *Foxholes and Color Lines: Desegregating the U.S. Armed Forces* (Baltimore, Md.: Johns Hopkins University Press, 1998): 253.

3. McCarthyism, which hit its peak in the early years of the 1950s, made conservative whites view any social progressive movement as communistic in nature. At its peak in 1954, Senator Joseph McCarthy accused even the army of harboring communist spies.

4. Dudziak, *Cold War Civil Rights;* and MacLean, *Freedom Is Not Enough.*

5. Darlene Clark Hine, William C. Hine, and Stanley Harrold, *African Americans: A Concise History* (Upper Saddle River, N.J.: Prentice Hall, 2004); and Dudziak, *Cold War Civil Rights,* chapters 3 and 4.

6. MacLean, *Freedom Is Not Enough*, 35.

7. Dudziak, *Cold War Civil Rights*, 11–13.

8. MacLean, *Freedom Is Not Enough*, chapter 2 and pp. 37–38.

9. Mershon and Schlossman, *Foxholes and Color Lines*, 274; Morris J. MacGregor, *Integration of the Armed Forces: 1940–1965* (Washington, D.C.: Center of Military History, 1981).

10. Williams, *Torchbearers of Democracy*, introduction; and Lentz-Smith, *Freedom Struggles.*

11. The Research and Development Corporation (RAND) is a nonprofit think tank that first formed to offer research and analyses to the United States Military. A RAND study, commissioned by the Clinton administration on the possible integration of gays in the military, used the integration of racial minorities as a case study. Study and updates available at http://www.rand.org/pubs/monographs/MG1056 .html (accessed on August 20, 2014); Mershon and Schlossman, *Foxholes and Color Lines*, 274.

12. Black representation in the military fluctuated throughout the 1950s and early 1960s. The army continued to have the largest proportion of African Americans serving, at about 13.7 percent of the total enlisted population in 1954. Mershon and Schlossman, *Foxholes and Color Lines*, 253 and 255.

13. Ibid., chapters 9–11.

14. Lillian Dunlap, *33 Years*, 86–87; and Bailey, *Autobiography*, 52–56.

15. Bailey, *Autobiography*, 104 and 123–24.

16. Mershon and Schlossman, *Foxholes and Color Lines*, 273.

17. Ibid., 275.

18. Although Eisenhower's 1957 battle in Little Rock, Arkansas, showed a reluctant willingness to enforce federal law in the name of national unity, with respect to the military and off-base race discrimination, government officials did little to enforce similar changes in the armed forces. This again revealed a reluctance to suggest or even promote the military as an organ for larger civilian social changes. Ibid., 252–53, 266–72, and 277.

19. Dudziak, *Cold War Civil Rights*, 155–57.

20. "Inaugural Address of President John F. Kennedy," January 20, 1961, Washington, D.C., transcript and video available at http://www.jfklibrary.org/Asset-Viewer/ BqXIEM9F4024ntFl7SVAjA.aspx (accessed August 20, 2014).

21. Although Kennedy's early presidency was fraught with one foreign affairs crisis after another, Kennedy could not ignore domestic race problems. He grew increasingly cognizant of the need to address race relations and by the time of his death supported civil rights legislation. However, race was not the only social issue on the president's radar. Increasing interest in women's rights positioned gender equality, albeit not on the same level as race equality, as another component to the search for human rights. In late 1961, Kennedy organized the President's Commission on the Status of Women. Kessler-Harris, *In Pursuit of Equity*, 213–15.

22. Hine, Hine, and Harrold, *African Americans*, 419–24.

23. Mershon and Schlossman, *Foxholes and Color Lines*, 274.

24. Ibid., 294; Morris J. MacGregor and Bernard C. Nalty, eds., *Blacks in the United States Armed Forces: Basic Documents*, vol. 13 (Wilmington, Del.: Scholarly Resources, 1977): 175; and MacGregor, *Integration*, 547–48.

25. Mershon and Schlossman, *Foxholes and Color Lines*, 295.

26. Given the postwar violence directed against returning African American veterans following World War II, these fears were well grounded.

27. Clara Adams-Ender, with Blair S. Walker, *My Rise to the Stars: How a Share-cropper's Daughter Became an Army General* (Lake Ridge, Va.: CAPE, 2001), 81–85.

28. MacGregor, *Integration*, 516; and Carl M. Brauer, *John F. Kennedy and the Second Reconstruction* (New York: Columbia University Press, 1977), 283–84.

29. Members of the NACGN participated in a November 1943 political strategy meeting of national black leaders. Their goals were to set an agenda concerning African Americans for President Roosevelt's upcoming reelection. See chapter 2 [herewith] and Records, NAACP, reel 2.

30. Margaret E. Bailey was the first African American nurse to hold the rank of lieutenant colonel (1964) and colonel (1970). Clara Adams-Ender was the second African American female nurse to become the ANC chief (1987). Both discuss their early experiences of serving in the military during the height of the civil rights movement. Bailey, *Autobiography*, 82–88 and 104–6; and Adams-Ender, *My Rise to the Stars*, 81–85.

31. The value of this order, according the Mershon and Schlossman, lay in its symbolism. It did not immediately affect housing, but it gave civil rights activists the sense that the Kennedy administration was willing to issue nondiscrimination measures to federal programs. Mershon and Schlossman, *Foxholes and Color Lines*, 284.

32. Dudziak, *Cold War Civil Rights*, chapter 6; Kessler-Harris, *In Pursuit of Equity*, 239–46; and Hine, Hine, and Harrold, *African Americans*, 424–27.

33. Margaret Culkin Banning, "Women in the Defense Decade," *American Journal of Nursing* 51, no. 12 (December 1951): 749.

34. Susan Hartmann, "Women's Employment and the Domestic Ideal in the Early Cold War Years," in Meyerowitz, *Not June Cleaver*, 84–100.

35. Senate Subcommittee on Labor or the Committee on Labor and Public Welfare, *Equal Pay Act of 1963: Hearings on S. 882 and S. 910*, 88th Congress, 1st session, 1963, 1–2.

36. The Intergroup Relations Committee, formed in 1948, attempted to improve relations between (racial, religious, gender) minority nurses and majority nurses and among the institutions, employers, and communities where nurses served. The ANC and the ANA had a long-established relationship that denoted the importance of the civilian nursing profession to military nursing, and vice versa.

37. "ANA Policies on Intergroup Relations," *American Journal of Nursing* 56, no. 2 (February 1956): 167; and Grace E. Marr, "Discrimination Is on Its Way Out: The

Nursing Profession Keeps Pace," *American Journal of Nursing* 56, no. 2 (February 1956): 166–68.

38. Gamble, *Making a Place for Ourselves*; and Carnegie, *Path We Tread*.

39. Grace Marr, "A Profession's Role in Integration," *American Journal of Nursing* 56, no. 11 (November 1956): 1403.

40. Shaw, *What a Woman*.

41. Hine, *Black Women in White*, ix; and Shaw, *What a Woman*.

42. Marr, "Profession's Role," 1403; and Marr, "Discrimination," 166–68.

43. Barbara G. Schutt, "Complacency or Leadership towards Integration," *American Journal of Nursing* 63, no.9 (September 1963): 69; and "Nurses March and Care for Marchers," *American Journal of Nursing* 63, no. 10 (October 1963): 76–77.

44. Leighow notes that married nurses were able to gain accommodations not yet available to women in other professions. This included "maternity leave and on-site childcare." Susan Rimby Leighow, "An Obligation to Participate: Married Nurses' Labor Force Participation in the 1950s," in Meyerowitz, *Not June Cleaver*, 37–56.

45. The official history of the U.S. Army Nurse Corps maintains that only minor problems occurred with respect to the integration effort during the Korean conflict. However, Captain Helen Dunne acknowledged that in those cases she believed that both nursing care and the performance of the officers suffered as a result. Helen I. Dunne to Ida Graham Price, May 21, 1954, ANCA, OSG.

46. In 1979 Hazel Johnson-Brown became the first African American female general in the Department of Defense. Carolyn M. Feller and Constance J. Moore, *Highlights in the History of the Army Nurse Corps* (Washington, D.C.: Center of Military History, 1995), 51.

47. Hazel Johnson-Brown, interviewed by Lt. Colonel Charles F. Bombard, February 16, 1984, Oral History Collection, ANCA, OSG, box 9.

48. Brown's race negotiation is similarly echoed by fellow officer Clara Adams-Ender, who remembers being told by another African American female nurse officer that she must be above reproach in her behavior regardless of how nonblacks act around her. Adams-Ender, *My Rise to the Stars*, 81–85.

49. Brown, "Oral History Interview," 43.

50. Ibid., 40–47.

51. Adams-Ender, *My Rise to the Stars*, 102–3.

52. LeRoy N. Craig, "Another Goal Achieved," *Nursing Outlook* (March 1956): 175–76; Sarnecky, *History*, 296–97.

53. Colonel Mildred I. Clark, interviewed by Lt. Col. Nancy R. Adams, 1986, vol. 1, transcript, ANCA, OSG, 165–66.

54. Frances P. Bolton to LeRoy Craig, February 19, 1958, Frances P. Bolton Papers, WRHS, folder 142.

55. C. G. Houser, interviewed by Cindy Houser, March 8, 1992, University of North Texas Oral History Collection, no. 874.

56. This is not to suggest that married men did not engage in homosexual behaviors or to suggest that gay men did not marry women; it is only to imply that married

male nurses often relieved some fears that male nurses were effeminate and most likely gay.

57. Leo LaBell, interviewed by Kara Vuic, Kara Dixon Vuic Collection, Vietnam Archive at Texas Tech University, p. 4 and p. 20; Robert J. Wehner, interviewed by Cindy Houser, August 22, 1992, University of North Texas Oral History Collection no. 940; and C. G. Houser, interviewed by C. Houser.

58. Wehner, interviewed by Houser, August 22, 1992, 2–3.

59. The army listed about 230 male reserve officers on concurrent active duty by mid-1959. Col. Margaret Harper, September 23, 1959, "Utilization of Male Army Nurse Corps Officers in AMEDS Activities," ANCA, OSG, Falls Church, Va., box 110 and box 125; and "Information as to Male Nurse Utilization as of 13 May 1959," Frances P. Bolton Papers, WRHS, folder 142.

60. LeRoy Craig to Frances P. Bolton, February 13, 1958, Frances P. Bolton Papers, WRHS, folder 142.

61. The military fully expected male nurses to have long-term career prospects, even though legislation prevented them from fully succeeding in the service. "Male Nurse Utilization Data (Army) As of 23 September 1959," Frances P. Bolton Papers, WRHS, folder 142.

62. Ibid.

63. LaBell, interviewed by Vuic, 5.

64. The commissioning of female physicians was under debate in 1950 at the same moment that male nurses legislation went before Congress. The commissioning of female doctors did not elicit the same passionate response as the commissioning of male nurses. Witt, Bellafaire, Granrud, and Binker, *Defense Weapon*, 132–34; and Morris A. Wolf, "Men Nurses in Services," *New York Times*, May 5, 1952.

65. Lt. Col. Alice M. Gritsavage quoted in Dorothy Brandon, "Calls Army Nurse 'Hazard to Troops,'" *Washington Post*, June 1, 1952; and Dorothy Brandon, "Men to Replace Nurses Up Front Urged by Korean Nurses' Leader," *New York Herald Tribune*, May 5, 1952.

66. Clark, interviewed by Adams, 168.

67. See chapter 3 herewith. In the U.S. Navy, pharmacists' mates had served this dual role since the early part of twentieth century. Male nurses, however, did not serve in the Navy Nurse Corps.

68. Originally, this training was open only to male nurses and would not be open to women for several years. Male nurses also served as part of medical detachments with special operations units; this was also an assignment open only to men. House of Representatives, "Authorizing Regular Commission for Male Nurses and Medical Specialists in the Army, Navy, and Air Force," 89th Congress, 2nd session, report 1823, August 9, 1966.

69. Feller and Moore, "Highlights in the History of the Army Nurse Corps," 29 and 31; Clark, interviewed by Adams, 169–170.

70. The lack of weapons training also precluded women from duty with the airborne division. Adams-Ender, *My Rise to the Stars*, 94.

71. Harper's emphasis on qualifications in assignments suggested a "fairness" view of duty. She later writes that it would appear discriminatory for one group to have hazardous duty all the time. While this is certainly part of her viewpoint, equally apparent was her attempt at sheltering women's position for the future. Harper, "Utilization of Male Army Nurse Corps Officers in AMEDS Activities."

72. H. W. Glattly to S. B. Hays, August 6, 1952, "Summary of Opinion Survey on Male Nurse Program," ANCA, OSG, box 110.

73. Army recruitment campaigns since World War II touted the great opportunities for advancement, job security, and travel for women in the Army Nurse Corps.

74. See chapter 4 herewith. "Gender-Male Nurses," ANCA, OSG, box 110a.

75. Leighow's study on the return and acceptance of married female nurses into the workforce shows that nursing shortages led to wider acceptance of working women in the 1950s. Leighow, "Obligation to Participate," 37–56.

76. The army instituted "Operation Nightingale" in February 1963 to stimulate public awareness of the army nurse and explain their need for nearly two thousand nurses. Kara Vuic notes that of the twenty-eight recruitment advertisements between 1963 and 1972, only one had pictures of either a male nurse or a black female nurse. Kara Dixon Vuic, "'Officer. Nurse. Women.': Army Nurse Corps Recruitment for the Vietnam War," *Nursing History Review* 14, no. 1 (September 2005): 118–120; "Army Is Facing a Critical Shortage of Nurses; Navy and Air Force Report a Different Picture," *Army, Navy, Air Force Journal and Register* (March 2, 1963): 10; and Feller and Moore, *Highlights*, 36.

77. African American female nurses already serving in the ANC made inroads in equality and better representation. In July 1964 Margaret E. Bailey was promoted to lieutenant colonel. Feller and Moore, *Highlights*, 38.

78. Col. Mildred I. Clark, October 16, 1964, "The Army Nurse Corps: Looking Ahead in 1965," ANCA, OSG.

79. Feller and Moore, *Highlights*, 37–38.

80. Leonard D. Heaton to Frances P. Bolton, May 22, 1961, Frances P. Bolton Papers, WRHS, folder 142; and "Background Information Concerning Professional Nursing and Male Nurses—Including Experience Data in AMEDS as of May 10, 1961," Frances P. Bolton Papers, WRHS, folder 142; and American Nurses' Association, "Facts about Nursing," 1960.

81. Heaton to Bolton, May 22, 1961.

82. Clark, "The Army Nurse Corps."

83. Bolton introduced H.R. 8135 in 1961 and H.R. 1034 in January 1963. They were identical bills, but both went nowhere in Congress. Clark, "Army Nurse Corps," 4.

84. Feller and Moore, *Highlights*, 28–29, and 39.

85. The drafted yielded 124 commissioned and 27 warrant officers for the ANC. Sarnecky, *History*, 339; and Feller and Moore, *Highlights*, 40.

86. House of Representatives, "Authorizing Regular Commission for Male Nurses and Medical Specialists in the Army, Navy, and Air Force," and Senate, "Authorizing

Regular Commission for Male Nurses and Medical Specialists in the Army, Navy, and Air Force," 89th Congress, 2nd session, report 1596, September 9 (legislative day September 7), 1966.

87. Frances P. Bolton introduced H.R. 420 in January 1966, and Samuel Stratton, a representative from New York, introduced identical legislation in May. Feller and Moore, *Highlights*, 40.

Conclusion

1. Col. Althea E. Williams to Jeanne M. Treacy, August 15, 1968, ANCA, OSG, box 110.

2. Colonel Capel to Lieutenant Colonel Nuttall, April 4, 1972, ANCA, OSG, box 110a.

3. Feller and Moore, *Highlights*, 41 and 43.

4. Sarnecky, *History*, 327–28; "U-BAD Newsletters," [1972?] Mary Sarnecky Collection, vols. 8 and 9, ANCA, OSG, box 88; and Kara Dixon Vuic, *Officer, Nurse, Woman: The Army Nurse Corps in the Vietnam War* (Baltimore, Md.: Johns Hopkins University Press, 2010).

5. Army Nurse Corps Newsletter, Historical Articles, "Proud to Serve: African American Army Nurse Corps Officers" and "Proud to Serve: The Evolution of Male Army Nurse Corps Officers"; and Mary Sarnecky, *A Contemporary History of the U.S. Army Nurse Corps* (Washington, D.C.: Borden Institute, 2010).

6. Erline W. Perkins, "The Registered Nurse: A Professional Person?" *American Journal of Nursing* 63, no. 2 (February 1963): 90–92.

7. Founded in 1974 as the National Male Nurses Association, in 1981 the group voted to change its name to the American Assembly for Men in Nursing.

8. Sarnecky, *Contemporary History*, and Army Nurse Corps Newsletter, Historical Articles, "Proud to Serve: African American Army Nurse Corps Officers" and "Proud to Serve: The Evolution of Male Army Nurse Corps Officers."

Selected Bibliography

Manuscript Collections

ARMY NURSE CORPS ARCHIVES, OFFICE OF THE SURGEON GENERAL, FALLS CHURCH, VA.

Box 1: Army Medical Department (AMEDD) History
Box 9: Hazel Johnson-Brown, Oral History
Box 13: Lt. Col. Mary Pitchard, Oral History
Box 28: Col. Florence A. Blanchfield, Bio File
Box 29: Col. Mildred I. Clark, Bio File
Box 79: Nursing Shortages
Box 108: African Americans—WWII
Box 109: Race—African Americans
Box 110: Gender—Male Nurses
Box 110a: Gender—Male Nurses
Box 111: Gender—DACOWITS
Box 115: Newsletters—Chiefs of the ANC
Box 125: History—ANC
Box 140: WWII—General History
Box 177: History—WWII Occupation 1946–47
Box 178: History—Korean War Correspondence

HOWARD GOTLIEB ARCHIVAL RESEARCH CENTER, BOSTON UNIVERSITY, BOSTON, MASS.

American Nurses' Association
Luther Christman Papers
Mary M. Roberts Papers

MARY SARNECKY COLLECTION—RESEARCH NOTES

Box 14: History of Male Nurses
Box 22: World War II History
Box 25: Mary Quinn—Mixed Blessings Poem
Box 88: Education, WRAIN Minority Students

MOORLAND-SPINGARN RESEARCH CENTER, HOWARD UNIVERSITY, WASHINGTON, D.C.

Mabel K. Staupers Papers
Howard University Men and Women in the Armed Forces 1941–1946
Vertical Files: "Nurses and Nursing"

SCHLESINGER LIBRARY, RADCLIFFE INSTITUTE, CAMBRIDGE, MASS.

Edith Nourse Rogers Papers

UNITED STATES NATIONAL ARCHIVES AND RECORDS ADMINISTRATION, COLLEGE PARK, MD.

Record Group 44: Records of the Office of Government Reports
Record Group 52: Records of the Bureau of Medicine and Surgery
Record Group 107: Records of the (Secretary of War) Office
Record Group 111: Records of the Chief Signal Officer
Record Group 112: Records of the Surgeon General (Army)
Record Group 160: Records of the Headquarters Armed Service Forces
Record Group 165: Records of the War Department and Special Staff
Record Group 200: Records of the American National Red Cross
Record Group 208: Records of the Office of War Information
Record Group 330: Records of the Office of the Secretary of Defense
Record Group 335: Records of the Office of the Secretary of the Army 1903–1991
Record Group 338: Records of the U.S. Army Operations, Tactical and Support
    Organization
Record Group 342: Records of the U.S. Air Force Commands
Record Group 407: Records of the Adjunct General

UNIVERSITY ARCHIVES, UNIVERSITY OF MINNESOTA, TWIN CITIES

Katherine Jane Densford Papers

WESTERN RESERVE HISTORICAL SOCIETY, CLEVELAND, OHIO

Frances P. Bolton Papers

Journals/Newspapers

American Journal of Nursing, 1900–1970
Army Info Digest
Army, Navy, Air Force Journal and Register, 1963
The Army Nurse, 1944–45
Army Nurse Week
Baltimore Afro-American, 1940–1955
Chicago Defender, 1930–1960
Crisis, 1925–1955
The Connection: Retired Army Nurse Corps Association
Graduate Nurses, 1940–1950
Journal of Advanced Nursing, 1910
Journal of Negro Education, 1932–1949
Medical News, 1888
The Military Surgeon, 1928
National News Bulletin: National Association of Colored
New York Amsterdam News, 1940–1945
New York Herald Tribune, 1952
New York Times, 1940–1955
Opportunity, 1934
Pittsburgh Courier, 1940–1949
PM, 1940–1945
Public Health Nurse, 1931
RN Magazine, 1950
Stars and Strips Magazine, 1945
The Trained Nurse and Hospital Review, 1945
Washington Post, 1940–1944

Sources on Microfilm

Records of the National Association of Colored Graduate Nurses, 1908–1951
Records of the National Association for the Advancement of Colored People
Part 9: Discrimination in the U.S. Armed Forces, 1918–1955
Part 15: Segregation and Discrimination—Complaints and Responses, 1940–1955
Part 18: Special Subjects, 1940–1955

Reports and Pamphlets

American Nurses' Association, "Committee on Legislation," 41st Convention, House
of Delegates Section Reports, 1956–1958.
American Nurses' Association. *Facts about Nursing*. Kansas City, Mo.: American
Nurses' Association, 1943.

American Nurses' Association. *Facts about Nursing.* Kansas City, Mo.: American Nurses' Association, 1946.

American Nurses' Association. *Facts about Nursing.* Kansas City, Mo.: American Nurses' Association, 1950.

American Nurses' Association. *Facts about Nursing.* Kansas City, Mo.: American Nurses' Association, 1960.

Brown, Esther Lucile. *Nursing for the Future: A Report Prepared for the National Nursing Council.* New York: Sage, 1948.

Clark, Colonel Mildred I. "The Army Nurse Corps: Looking Ahead in 1965." October 16, 1964.

Feller, Carolyn M., and Constance J. Moore, eds. *Highlights in the History of the Army Nurse Corps.* Washington D.C.: Center of Military History, United States Army, 1995.

Gallup, George H. *Gallup Poll—Public Opinion, 1949–1958,* vol. 2. New York: Random House, 1972.

Lawson, Steven, ed. *To Secure These Rights: The Report of Harry S. Truman's Committee on Civil Rights.* Boston: Bedford/St. Martin's, 2004.

Manning, Lory, and Vanessa R. Wight. *Women in the Military: Where They Stand.* Washington, D.C.: Women's Research and Education Institute, 2000.

National Association of Colored Graduate Nurses and the National Nursing Council for War Service. *Facts about Negro Nurses and the War.* New York: NACGN and NNCWS Headquarters, 1945.

Nightingale, Florence. *Notes on Nursing: What It Is, and What It Is Not.* 1859. Reprint. Philadelphia: Lippincott, 1992.

Unpublished Documents

Clark, Lt. Col. Mildred I. "Stand By for Korea, February 6, 1962." Army Nurse Corps Archives, Office of the Surgeon General.

Mattern, 1st Lt. Mary Jane. "Combat Nurse." Army Nurse Corps Archives, Office of the Surgeon General.

McIver, Pearl, Senior Nursing Consultant. "*Negro Nurses and the War Effort.*" U.S. Public Service for National Negro Health Week, April 1943. Mabel K. Staupers Collection, Moorland-Spingarn Research Center, Howard University, Washington, D.C., box 2.

Standlee, Mary, and Col. Florence Blanchfield. "The Appointment of Racial Minorities in the ANC, 1950 (?)." Army Nurse Corps Archives, Office of Surgeon General.

"War Neuroses Subcommittee Minutes." May 1, 1941. National Archives and Records Administration, RG 215.

Interview Collections

ARMY NURSE CORPS ARCHIVES, ORAL HISTORY COLLECTION

Mildred I. Clark

Hazel Johnson-Brown

UNIVERSITY OF NORTH TEXAS, ORAL HISTORY PROJECT

Tilliman E. Barrington, no. 989

Carl Horton, no. 1198

C. G. Houser, no. 874

Oscar Houser, no. 922

John Sherner, no. 953

Robert J. Wehner, no. 940

**KARA DIXON VUIC COLLECTION, VIETNAM ARCHIVE
AT TEXAS TECH UNIVERSITY**

Dick Berry

Leo LaBell

Barry Powell

John Sherner

Billy Storey

United States Government Documents

Public Health Service. *The United States Cadet Nurse Corps and Other Federal Nursing Training Programs 1943–48*. Washington, D.C.: U.S. Government Printing Office, 1950.

U.S. Congress. *Congressional Record*, March 5, 1945: 1729.

U.S. Congress. *Congressional Record*, May 20, 1954: 6547.

U.S. Congress, House of Representatives. "Authorizing Regular Commission for Male Nurses and Medical Specialists in the Army, Navy, and Air Force." 89th Congress, 2nd session, Report 1823, August 9, 1966.

U.S. Congress, House of Representatives. *Message from the President of the United States*. 79th Congress, 1st session, January 6, 1945, document 1, p. 7.

U.S. Congress, Senate. "Authorizing Regular Commission for Male Nurses and Medical Specialists in the Army, Navy, and Air Force." 89th Congress, 2nd session, Report 1596, September 9 (legislative day September 7), 1966.

Online Resources

American Nurses Association. "Basic Historical Review." American Nurses Association. Available at http://nursingworld.org/FunctionalMenuCategories/AboutANA/History (accessed August 20, 2014).

"Inaugural Address of President John F. Kennedy." January 20, 1961. Washington, D.C. Transcript and video available at http://www.jfklibrary.org/Asset-Viewer/ BqXIEM9F4024ntFl7SVAjA.aspx (accessed August 20, 2014).

Roosevelt, Franklin D. "Four Freedoms Speech." Annual Message to Congress. January 1941. Franklin D. Roosevelt Presidential Library and Museum. Available at http://www.fdrlibrary.marist.edu/pdfs/ffreadingcopy.pdf (accessed on August 10, 2014).

Truman, Harry S. "Special Message to Congress." February 2, 1948. Digital Collection: Truman Presidential Library. Available at http://trumanlibrary.org/publicpapers/ index.php?pid=1380 (accessed August 20, 2014).

Published Materials

Adams-Ender, Clara, with Blair S. Walker. *My Rise to the Stars: How a Sharecropper's Daughter Became an Army General.* Lake Ridge, Va: CAPE, 2001.

Apel, Otto F., and Pat Apel. *MASH: An Army Surgeon in Korea.* Lexington: University Press of Kentucky, 1988.

Bailey, Col. Margaret F. *The Challenge: Autobiography of Colonel Margaret F. Bailey.* Lisle, Ill.: Tucker, 1999.

Brown, Harvey E. *The Medical Department of the United States Army 1775–1873.* Washington, D.C.: Surgeon General's Office, 1873.

Dunlap, Lillian. *33 Years of Army Nursing: An Interview with Brigadier General Lillian Dunlap.* Conducted by Cynthia A. Gurney. Washington, D.C.: U.S. Army Nurse Corps, 2001.

Horwitz, Dorothy G., ed., *We Will Not Be Strangers: Korean War Letters between a M.A.S.H. Surgeon and His Wife.* Urbana: University of Illinois Press, 1997.

Lee, Ulysses. *The Employment of Negro Troops.* Washington, D.C.: Office of the Chief of Military History, United States Army, 1966.

MacGregor, Morris J. *Integration of the Armed Forces 1940–1965.* Defense Studies Series. Washington, D.C.: Center of Military History, United States Army, 1981.

———, and Bernard C. Nalty, eds., *Blacks in the United States Armed Forces: Basic Documents*, vol. 13. Wilmington, Del.: Scholarly Resources, 1977.

Nightingale, Florence. *Notes on Nursing: What It Is, and What It Is Not.* 1859. Reprint. Philadelphia: Lippincott, 1992.

Smith, Clarence McKittrick. *The Medical Department: Hospitalization and Evacuation, Zone of the Interior.* The U.S. Army in WWII: The Technical Services. Washington, D.C.: Center of Military History, United States Army, 1956.

Staupers, Mabel K. *No Time for Prejudice: A Story of the Integration of Negroes in Nursing in the United States.* New York: Macmillan, 1961.

Index

Adams-Ender, Clara, 113–14, 119, 179n30, 180n48

African American nurses: and the ANA, 30, 32–33, 57, 85, 147n56, 152n34, 155n55; challenges to racial ideologies, 5, 9; and the civil rights movement, 28–35; duty of professionals as role models, 116; Korean War, 98; letters detailing experiences, 47–49, 157n111; male nurses, 55, 72–73, 85, 146n44; nurse training schools, 22–23, 30, 147n55, 151nn24–25, 153n48, 171n41; overseas placement of, 156n96, 157n110; POW camps, 47–49; professional organizations (*see also* ANA above), 57, 132, 152n34; professionalization of, 27, 29–35; public acceptance of, 77–78; quotas, 40–42, 93, 167n95; real *vs.* symbolic changes, 117–27; and the Red Cross, 28; and social justice activities, 113–14; Spanish American War, 21; World War I, 23–24, 28, 38–39; World War II, 81–82. *See also* Army Nurse Corps; nurse shortages

African Americans: black regiments, 155n71; healthcare for soldiers, 45–46; integration of the military, 83–84, 107, 109, 174n79, 178nn11–12, 178n18; Korean War, 97–98; necessary negotiations, 118–19, 180n48; nurse shortages, 30; post-war role of, 82; separate but equal doctrine, 37–46, 81, 108–9

Agnew, W. J. C., 75

airborne training, 122, 181n68

Alexian Brothers, 15, 19, 144–45n26

American Assembly for Men in Nursing, 132

American Association of Industrial Nurses, 174n83

American Association of Nurse Anesthetists, 96

American Dilemma, An (Mrydal), 169n16

American Federation of Labor, 51

American Hospital Association: on male nurses, 72–73

American Journal of Nursing: about, 161n19; on African American nurses during World War II, 40; on duty of professionals as role models, 116; on male nurses, 57, 59, 63, 72; on nurse shortages, 46

American Nurses' Association (ANA): and access to healthcare, 79, 116; African American nurses, 30, 32–33, 57, 85, 147n56, 152n34, 155n55; and ANC, 22; antidiscrimination campaign, 4, 85; Economic Security Program, 116; gender equity, 87–104; gender ideology, 56–59; incorporation of NACGN members, 87, 114, 132; Intergroup Relations Committee, 84–85, 170nn31–32, 179–80n36; Joint Committee on Nursing in National Security, 96, 174n83; and male nurses, 63, 67, 71–73, 85, 87, 146n44; membership requirements, 161n12, 161n18, 171n40;

Vietnam War, 9, 114, 126–27, 177n126
Vinson, Carl, 94
violence, racial, 82, 169n15
Vuic, Kara Dixon, 125, 182n76

Walter Reed Army Hospital, 118
Walter Reed Army Institute of Nursing, 9, 131
war, 3, 21–22. See also *specific wars*
War Department: African American nurses, 76; male nurses, 64–66, 71–78; nursing shortages, 74; racial discrimination, 25–26; separate but equal doctrine, 37–46. *See also* Defense Department
Washington, Booker T., 29, 152n38
weapons training, 122, 182n70
Welch, John, 69
White, Walter, 1–2, 35–36, 154n62, 157n100
White Citizens' Councils, 108
Williams, Chad, 151n20
Williams, Christine, 55
Wilson, Woodrow, 70

Witte, Frances, 59–60
Wolf, Morris, 102
women doctors, 94, 102, 176n112
Women's Armed Services Integration Act (1948), 168n8
Women's Army Corps, 73
Women's Medical Specialist Corps, 173n72
women's rights movement, 114–15
Wood, Casey, 10–11
Wooding, Nathaniel, 64
World War I, 23–24, 28, 38–39, 64, 163–64n47
World War II: African American nurses, 81–82; capture of female nurses, 176n104; Executive Order 8802 (1941), 41; gender and racial ideologies, 3–4; integration campaigns, 7–8, 37–52; male nurses, 64–69, 71–78; mobilization propaganda, 160n2; nursing shortages, 25–26, 43–52, 74, 166n85

yellow fever, 21, 146–47n48

CHARISSA J. THREAT is an assistant professor of history at Spelman College.

WOMEN IN AMERICAN HISTORY

Women Doctors in Gilded-Age Washington: Race, Gender, and Professionalization
  Gloria Moldow
Friends and Sisters: Letters between Lucy Stone and Antoinette Brown Blackwell,
  1846–93   *Edited by Carol Lasser and Marlene Deahl Merrill*
Reform, Labor, and Feminism: Margaret Dreier Robins and the Women's Trade
  Union League   *Elizabeth Anne Payne*
Private Matters: American Attitudes toward Childbearing and Infant Nurture
  in the Urban North, 1800–1860   *Sylvia D. Hoffert*
Civil Wars: Women and the Crisis of Southern Nationalism   *George C. Rable*
I Came a Stranger: The Story of a Hull-House Girl   *Hilda Satt Polacheck;
  edited by Dena J. Polacheck Epstein*
Labor's Flaming Youth: Telephone Operators and Worker Militancy, 1878–1923
  Stephen H. Norwood
Winter Friends: Women Growing Old in the New Republic, 1785–1835   *Terri L. Premo*
Better Than Second Best: Love and Work in the Life of Helen Magill
  Glenn C. Altschuler
Dishing It Out: Waitresses and Their Unions in the Twentieth Century
  Dorothy Sue Cobble
Natural Allies: Women's Associations in American History   *Anne Firor Scott*
Beyond the Typewriter: Gender, Class, and the Origins of Modern American
  Office Work, 1900–1930   *Sharon Hartman Strom*
The Challenge of Feminist Biography: Writing the Lives of Modern American Women
  Edited by Sara Alpern, Joyce Antler, Elisabeth Israels Perry, and Ingrid Winther Scobie
Working Women of Collar City: Gender, Class, and Community in Troy,
  New York, 1864–86   *Carole Turbin*
Radicals of the Worst Sort: Laboring Women in Lawrence, Massachusetts, 1860–1912
  Ardis Cameron
Visible Women: New Essays on American Activism   *Edited by Nancy A. Hewitt
  and Suzanne Lebsock*
Mother-Work: Women, Child Welfare, and the State, 1890–1930   *Molly Ladd-Taylor*
Babe: The Life and Legend of Babe Didrikson Zaharias   *Susan E. Cayleff*
Writing Out My Heart: Selections from the Journal of Frances E. Willard, 1855–96
  Edited by Carolyn De Swarte Gifford
U.S. Women in Struggle: A *Feminist Studies* Anthology   *Edited by
  Claire Goldberg Moses and Heidi Hartmann*
In a Generous Spirit: A First-Person Biography of Myra Page   *Christina Looper Baker*
Mining Cultures: Men, Women, and Leisure in Butte, 1914–41   *Mary Murphy*
Gendered Strife and Confusion: The Political Culture of Reconstruction
  Laura F. Edwards
The Female Economy: The Millinery and Dressmaking Trades, 1860–1930
  Wendy Gamber